Get Through

MRCPsych: MCQs for Paper 2

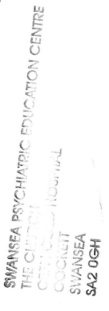

Get Through
MRCPsych: MCQs for Paper 2

Arunraj Kaimal MBBS MRCPsych
Consultant Old Age Psychiatrist and Honorary Lecturer in Psychiatry,
Wythenshawe Hospital, Manchester, UK

Manoj Rajagopal MBBS MRCPsych MSc
ST-5 in Old Age Psychiatry, Hope Hospital, Manchester, UK

Salman Karim MBBS FCPS MSc
Consultant Old Age Psychiatrist and Honorary Lecturer in Psychiatry,
Hope Hospital, Manchester, UK

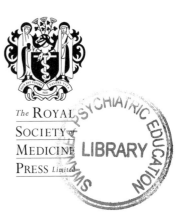

The ROYAL
SOCIETY of
MEDICINE LIBRARY
PRESS Limited

© 2009 Royal Society of Medicine Press Ltd

Published by the Royal Society of Medicine Press Ltd
1 Wimpole Street, London W1G 0AE, UK
Tel: +44 (0)20 7290 2921
Fax: +44 (0)20 7290 2929
Email: publishing@rsm.ac.uk
Website: www.rsmpress.co.uk

British Library Cataloguing in Publication Data
A catalogue record for this book is available from the British Library

ISBN: 978-1-85315-853-7

Distribution in Europe and Rest of World:
Marston Book Services Ltd
PO Box 269
Abingdon
Oxon OX14 4YN, UK
Tel: +44 (0)1235 465500
Fax: +44 (0)1235 465555
Email: direct.order@marston.co.uk

Distribution in the USA and Canada:
Royal Society of Medicine Press Ltd
c/o BookMasters Inc
30 Amberwood Parkway
Ashland, OH 44805, USA
Tel: +1 800 247 6553/+1 800 266 5564
Fax: +1 419 281 6883
Email: order@bookmasters.com

Distribution in Australia and New Zealand:
Elsevier Australia
30-52 Smidmore Street
Marrickville NSW 2204, Australia
Tel: +61 2 9517 8999
Fax: +61 2 9517 2249
Email: service@elsevier.com.au

Typeset by Techset Composition Limited, Salisbury, UK
Printed and bound in Great Britain by Bell & Bain, Glasgow

Contents

Introduction

The examination

The new MRCPsych examination consists of three written papers and one clinical examination (the CASC). There have been major changes to the format of the examination recently, the most important being the change from individual statement questions (ISQs) and extended matching items (EMIs) to 'best answer 1 of 5' style multiple choice questions (MCQs) and EMIs. Although there are a number of ISQ and EMI books available on the market, there are very few dedicated solely to the new-format 'best answer 1 of 5' MCQs.

In this book we have attempted to overcome this shortfall by providing 350 MCQs covering all areas of the MRCPsych Paper 2 curriculum. The presentation of questions in this book according to the subheadings in the new curriculum will make revision easier, making this book an essential companion for trainees preparing for the MRCPsych Paper 2 examination.

As described in the curriculum, each MCQ comprises a question stem, which is usually one or two sentences long but may be longer. The question stem is followed by a list of five options; candidates should choose the single option that best fits the question stem.

The MRCPsych Paper 2 examination is 3 hours long and contains 200 questions. Approximately one-third of the examination will be the EMI component. Candidates are advised to attempt all questions. No marks are deducted for incorrect answers. One mark is given for the correct answer.

Revising for the examination

The topics included in the Paper 2 examination are neurosciences, psychopharmacology, genetics, epidemiology, and advanced psychological processes and treatments. Knowledge of the latest developments in these fields is tested in the Paper 2 examination and hence candidates are advised to use the latest editions of textbooks for revision. In addition to this, they are advised to be familiar with the topics covered in the review articles (over the 12–18-month period before the examination) in the Royal College of Psychiatrists' journal *Advances in Psychiatric Treatment*, and editorials and review articles in the *British Journal of Psychiatry*. The journal *Evidence-Based Mental Health* (*EBMH*) gives summaries of a selection of the best studies from over 50 leading international medical journals. In *EBMH* the key details of each chosen study are presented in an informative abstract with an additional expert commentary on its clinical application. Since *EBMH* is published quarterly candidates are advised to go through the abstracts from the last eight publications before their examination.

One of the keys to examination success is to practise MCQs in the subject areas that regularly appear in the examination. We have covered all such areas in this book and provide a list of books useful in revision as well as the essential reference textbooks. We have used these books for reference in writing this MCQ book.

The best way to practise MCQs is in a group of candidates for the examination. In small groups, the recommended practice method is to solve MCQs by reading around the topic, and then compare the answers and explanations given in the book. It is important to remember that this book is not a substitute for standard textbooks and should be used as a guide to focus on important examination topics. In this book we have not included page numbers of textbooks within the answers. Candidates are expected to read around the topics covered in the MCQ stem from the suggested textbooks and further reading references detailed at the end of the answer section.

In the later part of revision, a few weeks before the examination, this book should be used as a practice examination, and 17 or 18 questions from each chapter should be solved in 2 hours (altogether 120 questions in one sitting), since the actual examination is 3 hours long and two-thirds of it consists of MCQs. Choosing different sets of multiples of 17 or 18 each time (for example, question numbers 1–17 from each chapter for the first practice examination and 18–34 for the second) will give the trainee the opportunity to undertake at least two practice examinations before the actual examination. Good time management is an important contributor to success and strict time keeping is essential in preparation for the examination.

It is also important to read and understand each stem thoroughly since some common terms used in MCQs may guide you to the correct response. Although there is no strict rule that any term indicates that the statement is true or false, the use of terms such as 'may', 'may be', 'can occur', 'can be', etc, could indicate an increased chance of the statement being true. Similarly, terms such as 'always occur' and 'never occur' could indicate the possibility of the statement being false.

Other terms such as 'characteristic', 'pathognomonic', 'common' and 'rare' should also be interpreted cautiously. Generally, 'characteristic' means that without the presence of that feature the diagnosis is doubtful; a 'pathognomonic' feature is found only in that condition; 'common' generally means found in more than 30%; and 'rare' means found in less than 5%.

We recommend working through the chapters of this book as early as possible before the examination date, reading around the topics given in a question stem from the books provided in the reading list and making notes for reference a few weeks before the examination. We suggest that you attempt the questions before checking the answers and any questions answered incorrectly should be noted and revised carefully in the weeks just before the examination. In this way we hope this book will be useful for consolidating your knowledge and helping you to get through the MRCPsych Paper 2 examination.

Arunraj Kaimal
Manoj Rajagopal
Salman Karim

Recommended reading

Preparation for the Paper 2 examination

British National Formulary. *BNF 57*. London: Pharmaceutical Press. Also available at: www.bnf.org/bnf.

Buckley P, Prewette D, Bird J, Harrison G. *Examination Notes in Psychiatry*, 4th edn. London: Hodder Education, 2004.

Gelder M, Harrison P, Cowen P. *Shorter Oxford Textbook of Psychiatry*, 5th edn. Oxford: Oxford University Press, 2006.

Hodges JR. *Cognitive Assessment for Clinicians*, 2nd edn. Oxford: Oxford University Press, 2007.

ICD-10: *The ICD-10 Classification of Mental and Behavioural Disorders: Clinical Descriptions and Diagnostic Guidelines*. Geneva: World Health Organization, 1990.

Munafo M. *Psychology for the MRCPsych*, 2nd edn. London: Hodder Education, 2002.

Oyebode F. *Sims' Symptoms in the Mind: An Introduction to Descriptive Psychopathology*, 4th edn. London: Saunders, 2008.

Puri B, Hall A. *Revision Notes in Psychiatry*, 2nd edn. London: Arnold/Hodder Education, 2004.

Sadock BJ, Sadock VA. *Kaplan and Sadock's Synopsis of Psychiatry*, 10th edn. Baltimore, MD: Lippincott Williams and Wilkins, 2008.

Smith EE, Bem DJ, Nolen-Hoeksema S. Chapters 2–6. In: *Atkinson and Hilgard's Introduction to Psychology*, 14th edn. Florence, KY: Wadsworth Publishing Company, 2003.

Taylor D, Paton C, Kerwin R. *Maudsley Prescribing Guidelines*, 9th edn. London: Informa Healthcare, 2007.

Wright P, Stern J, Phelan M. *Core Psychiatry*, 2nd edn. London: Saunders, 2005.

General revision

David A, Fleminger S, Kopelman M, Lovestone S, Mellers J. *Lishman's Organic Psychiatry: A Textbook of Neuropsychiatry*, 4th edn. Chichester: Wiley-Blackwell, 2009.

Fish FJ, Casey PR, Kelly B. *Fish's Clinical Psychopathology: Signs and Symptoms in Psychiatry*, 3rd edn. London: Royal College of Psychiatrists Publications, 2007.

Gross R. *Psychology: The Science of Mind and Behaviour*, 5th edn. London: Hodder Education, 2005.

Kumar P, Clark M. *Kumar and Clark's Clinical Medicine*, 7th edn. London: Saunders, 2009.

Stahl SM. *Stahl's Essential Psychopharmacology: Neuroscientific Basis and Practical Applications*, 3rd edn. Cambridge: Cambridge University Press, 2008.

1) Which of the following is true of prosopagnosia?

   a. It is the inability to recognize faces
   b. The recognition of other environmental objects is also usually impaired
   c. It is thought to result from disconnection of the left inferior temporal cortex from the left frontal lobe
   d. It is the same as associative visual agnosia
   e. It usually occurs early on in frontotemporal dementia

2) All of the following statements are true about disorders of visual perception, except:

   a. Apperceptive visual agnosia results from bilateral lesions in the visual association areas
   b. Colour perception may be ablated in lesions of the dominant occipital lobe
   c. Colour agnosia is the inability to name a colour despite the ability to point to it
   d. Central achromatopsia is a complete inability to perceive colour
   e. Simultanagnosia is the inability to integrate a visual scene to perceive it as a whole

3) Balint's syndrome includes all of the following, except:

   a. Failure to acknowledge blindness
   b. Optic ataxia
   c. Oculomotor apraxia
   d. Simultanagnosia
   e. Bilateral lesion in the occipitoparietal area

4) Gerstmann's syndrome includes all of the following, except:

   a. Agraphia
   b. Acalculia
   c. Finger agnosia
   d. Right–left disorientation
   e. Dominant temporal lobe lesions

5) Regarding the auditory system, which of the following is true?

    a. Sound localization is mediated by the dominant hemisphere in the brain

    b. Lexical processing is done in the right temporal lobe

    c. The syndrome of word deafness may reflect damage to the left parietal cortex

    d. The syndrome of auditory sound agnosia is the inability to recognize verbal sounds

    e. All of the above

6) Which of the following apraxias is correctly paired with its lesion or lesion site?

    a. Limb-kinetic apraxia—Supplementary motor area

    b. Ideomotor apraxia—Disconnection of Wernicke's area from the motor region

    c. Ideomotor apraxia—Left premotor area

    d. Ideational apraxia—Prefrontal cortex

    e. All of the above

7) Regarding clinical syndromes of language impairment, all of the following are true, except:

    a. In pure word deafness, the patient can speak fluently and virtually without error and can write normally

    b. In pure word blindness, the patient can describe or copy letters even though he or she cannot recognize them

    c. In pure word dumbness, the patient can repeat the words heard and can read aloud

    d. In pure agraphia, comprehension of written and spoken material is normal and the patient's own speech is unimpaired

    e. In pure word blindness, the patient can write spontaneously and to dictation

8) In Wernicke's dysphasia, all of the following are true, except:

    a. There is defective appreciation of the meaning of words

    b. Paraphrasic errors and neologisms are frequent

    c. Errors of grammar and syntax occur

    d. Faulty, non-fluent speech is produced with effort

    e. Normal rhythm and inflection are preserved and there are no articulatory defects

9) Which of the following is true of Broca's dysphasia?

    a. It is also known as receptive dysphasia

    b. Writing is not affected

    c. Normal rhythm and inflection are preserved

    d. The patient is clearly under stress while trying to speak

    e. The patient cannot usually recognize his or her mistakes

10) Regarding intelligence tests, all of the following are true, except:

a. Alfred Binet introduced the concept of mental age
b. The Wechsler Adult Intelligence Scale (WAIS) comprises 11 subtests made up of six verbal subtests and five performance subtests
c. On the WAIS, the simplest level of brain damage may be reflected in discrepancies between the verbal and performance IQs
d. The performance subtests in the WAIS include digit span
e. Visuoperception, somatoperception and manual dexterity are tested in object assembly tests in performance subtests of the WAIS

11) Regarding the National Adult Reading Test, all of the following statements are true, except:

a. It is suitable for estimating premorbid intelligence
b. It may also be used to estimate premorbid levels of verbal fluency
c. In patients with dementia of moderate severity, it may yield an underestimate of premorbid competence
d. It is more suitable for estimating premorbid intelligence than the Schonell test
e. It is a culture-free test

12) Which of the following is used as a rapid device for estimating performance IQ?

a. Raven's Progressive Matrices
b. The Bender-Gestalt Test
c. The Visual Object and Space Perception Battery
d. The Behavioural Inattention Test
e. The Token Test

13) Regarding memory tests, which of the following statements is true?

a. The Kendrick Object Learning Test is very stressful and less acceptable to elderly patients
b. Performance on the Benton Visual Retention Test correlates highly with intelligence and chronological age
c. Patients with dominant temporal lobe damage show major impairment with the Rey–Osterrieth Test
d. On the revised version of the Wechler Memory Scale, practice effects can be avoided if testing is repeated
e. A shortened version of the Rivermead Behavioural Memory Test, used with aphasic patients, has been shown to be sensitive to the effects of language impairment rather than memory deficits

14) All of the following tests are good indicators of frontal lobe function, except:

a. Tests of Verbal Fluency
b. Wisconsin Card Sorting Test
c. Stroop Test
d. Mini Mental State Examination
e. Cognitive Estimates Test

15) Which of the following is true of the Halstead–Reitan Battery?

    a. It can indicate whether brain damage is focal or diffuse
    b. It contains a category test
    c. It includes detailed assessments of the accuracy of sensory perception on each side of the body
    d. It tests finger recognition, graphaesthesia and stereognosis
    e. All of the above

16) Regarding dementia assessment, all of the following statements are true, except:

    a. The Blessed Dementia Scale is administered to the patient
    b. The Mini Mental State Examination is shown to discriminate well between patients with dementia and delirium
    c. The Geriatric Mental State Schedule covers the period of a month prior to examination
    d. The CAMCOG is specifically engineered to be user friendly for non-psychologists
    e. DEMQOL is a computer program derived from the Geriatric Mental State Schedule that arrives at levels of confidence for diagnosing organic brain syndrome, schizophrenia, depression, etc.

17) Regarding objective measures of personality in adults, which of the following statements is true?

    a. The Minnesota Multiphasic Personality Inventory (MMPI) does not emphasize major psychopathology
    b. The 16 Personality Factor Questionnaire has limited usefulness with clinical populations
    c. The Personality Assessment Inventory (PAI) does not include measures of psychopathology
    d. The California Personality Inventory (CPI) is well accepted as a diagnostic tool in a clinical population
    e. The Eysenck Personality Questionnaire (EPQ) is regarded as a very useful clinical diagnostic tool

18) Which of the following scales is useful in establishing the severity of illness and monitoring the treatment response?

    a. The Hamilton Rating Scale for Depression
    b. The Hamilton Anxiety Scale
    c. The Yale–Brown Obsessive Compulsive Scale
    d. The Structural Clinical Interview for DSM-IV Dissociative Disorders (SCID-D)
    e. All of the above

19) The Minnesota Multiphasic Personality Inventory (MMPI) validity scale contains:

a. A lie scale
b. An infrequency scale
c. A suppressor scale
d. All of the above
e. None of the above

20) The Minnesota Multiphasic Personality Inventory (MMPI) clinical scales include all of the following, except:

a. A depression scale
b. A phobia scale
c. A masculinity–femininity scale
d. A hysteria scale
e. A social introversion scale

21) Regarding projective measures of personality, all of the following are true, except:

a. The Rorschach Test is the most widely used and best-researched projective device
b. There is no generally accepted scoring system for the Thematic Apperception Test and it is time consuming
c. The Sentence Completion Test is lengthy in administration time, and not useful in clinical interviews
d. In the Holtzman Inkblot Technique, only one response is allowed per card
e. The Make-a-Picture-Story Test provides idiographic personality information through thematic analysis

22) All neuropsychological deficits are associated mainly with left hemisphere damage, except:

a. Aphasia
b. Right–left disorientation
c. Finger agnosia
d. Anosognosia
e. Limb apraxia

23) Which of the following statements is true of the Luria–Nebraska Neuropsychological Battery?

a. A children's version is available for use with 8- to 12-year-olds
b. The test is extremely sensitive in identifying problems like dyslexia and dyscalculia
c. It helps to localize the various cortical zones that are involved in a particular function
d. It is useful in establishing left or right cerebral dominance
e. All of the above

24) Regarding attitudes, all of the following statements are true, except:

   a. A semantic differential scale is used to measure attitude
   b. A five-point Likert scale is more sensitive in measuring attitudes than the dichotomous Thurstone Scale
   c. The scapegoat theory of prejudice explains an ego-defensive function in which the person blames the outgroup for personal and social problems
   d. In general, attitudes tend to predict behaviour if the individual is not aware of his or her attitudes
   e. When a person's behaviours are inconsistent with his or her attitudes, cognitive dissonance leads the person to change these attitudes

25) All of the following are objective tests of personality, except:

   a. The Myers–Briggs Inventory
   b. The Eysenck Personality Questionnaire
   c. The Hostility and Direction of Hostility Questionnaire
   d. The Q-Sort Test
   e. The Sentence Completion Test

26) Gardner's seven intelligences include all of the following, except:

   a. Linguistic intelligence
   b. Procedural intelligence
   c. Musical intelligence
   d. Bodily–kinaesthetic intelligence
   e. Intrapersonal intelligence

27) Regarding theories of intelligence, all of the following are true, except:

   a. Gardner's theory explains that the wide variety of adult roles found in different cultures cannot be explained by a single underlying intelligence
   b. Anderson's theory explains the existence of a basic processing mechanism and specific processors for propositional thought and visual and spatial functioning
   c. According to Sternberg's theory, differences in experience affect the ability to solve a given problem
   d. Ceci's bioecological theory rejects the idea of single general capacity for abstract problem solving
   e. According to Spearman's theory, factor s is the major determinant of performance on intelligence tests

28) Regarding errors of assessment, which of the following statements is true?

   a. The Hawthorne effect occurs when the presence of an interviewer influences the response
   b. The halo effect describes selecting answers to fit with other responses
   c. Response set is a tendency always to agree or disagree with questions
   d. Leniency error is a tendency to select extreme responses
   e. All of the above

29) Which of the following statements is true of IQ?

   a. It is the ratio of mental age to chronological age
   b. It has a normal distribution with a mean of 120 and a standard deviation of 15
   c. There is a natural increase in intellectual ability with age
   d. Performance IQ falls off with age more quickly than verbal IQ
   e. Neither Stanford–Binet nor Wechsler scales are useful as predictors of achievement in school

30) Regarding the validity of a test, all of the following statements are true, except:

   a. Predictive validity determines the extent of agreement between a present measurement and one in the future
   b. Concurrent validity compares the measure being assessed with an external valid yardstick at the same time
   c. Incremental validity refers to predictive validity and concurrent validity together
   d. Divergent validity is established when measures discriminate successfully between other measures of unrelated constructs
   e. Construct validity is determined by establishing both convergent and divergent validity

31) All of the following statements about the Present State Examination are true, except:

   a. It is available in at least 35 languages, and has been widely used in many countries
   b. It is a structured interview retaining the features of a clinical examination
   c. It identifies abnormal phenomena that have been present during a defined period of time
   d. It rates the severity of abnormal phenomena identified
   e. It is not very useful in research, especially for the assessment of severe mental illness

32) Which of the following statements is true about the Schedules for Clinical Assessment in Neuropsychiatry (SCAN)?

   a. They can be used to diagnose eating, somatoform, substance abuse and cognitive disorders
   b. They have four possible ratings
   c. They are compatible with PSE-9
   d. They allow ICD-10 and DSM-IV diagnoses
   e. All of the above

33) The International Personality Disorder Examination (IPDE):

   a. Does not assess phenomenology and life experiences
   b. Establishes psychiatric diagnosis according to DSM-IV
   c. Is an instrument comprising 153 closed questions
   d. Includes questions to determine frequency and duration
   e. Does not try to establish age of onset

34) All of the following statements about standardized assessment tools are true, except:

   a. The Diagnostic Interview Schedule (DIS) was used in the Epidemiological Catchment Area (ECA) project
   b. The Structured Clinical Interview Schedule (SCID) is available as a patient edition for use in the clinical population and as a non-patient edition for use in epidemiological studies
   c. The Composite International Diagnostic Interview (CIDI) provides ICD-10 and DSM-IV diagnoses
   d. CATEGO is a computer program based on SCID
   e. In Diagnostic Interview Schedule (DIS), disorders occurring at any time in a person's life are taken into account

35) All of the following statements are true about instruments for measuring symptoms, except:

   a. The Hamilton Anxiety Scale (HAS) is designed for rating anxiety in other disorders
   b. The Clinical Anxiety Scale is developed from the HAS, but focuses more on the symptoms of anxiety by leaving out depressive and somatic symptoms
   c. The Hamilton Rating Scale for Depression (HRSD) measures the severity of the depressive syndrome rather than the symptoms of depression
   d. The Beck Depression Inventory (BDI) is usually completed by the patient
   e. On the Montgomery–Åsberg Depression Rating Scale (MADRS), only psychological symptoms of depression are rated by an interviewer

36) The Positive and Negative Syndrome Scale (PANSS) rates:

    a. Blunted affect
    b. Emotional withdrawal
    c. Poor rapport
    d. Difficulty in abstract and stereotyped thinking
    e. All of the above

37) Which of the following is true of the General Health Questionnaire?

    a. It is designed as a screening instrument in primary care
    b. The full version can be completed in 10 minutes
    c. The full version contains 60 questions
    d. The total score indicates overall severity, expressed as whether a psychiatrist would judge the patient as a 'case' or a 'non-case'
    e. All of the above

38) A 58-year-old man with frontal lobe dementia starts to scribble on your table using your pen that was lying on it; when distracted from that he takes your spectacles from the table and puts them on. This behaviour is described as:

    a. Wartenberg's reflex
    b. Witzelsucht
    c. Utilization behaviour
    d. Perseveration
    e. Magnetic syndrome

39) A 64-year-old man with a history of left-sided parieto-occipital infarct can appreciate details of individual components of a complex picture but fails to understand the overall meaning of the picture. This phenomenon is known as:

    a. Visual object agnosia
    b. Prosopagnosia
    c. Simultanagnosia
    d. Anosognosia
    e. Gerstmann's syndrome

40) A 68-year-old man with previous left-sided cerebral infarct is unable to point to or name any of his body parts when asked. This condition is known as:

    a. Prosopagnosia
    b. Hemiasomatognosia
    c. Autotopagnosia
    d. Microsomatognosia
    e. Autoscopy

41) A patient with early dementia is unable to carry out the coordinated sequences of actions when he is asked to take a match from a box and light it by striking. This is an example of:

a. Limb-kinetic apraxia
b. Ideomotor apraxia
c. Ideational apraxia
d. Constructional apraxia
e. Utilization behaviour

42) The Cambridge Examination for Mental Disorders of the Elderly (CAMDEX) incorporates:

a. The Mini Mental State Examination
b. The Blessed Dementia Rating Scale
c. The Hachinski Ischaemic Score
d. CAMCOG
e. All of the above

43) Which of the following is true of the Mini Mental State Examination?

a. It covers the basic cognitive functions
b. It is a diagnostic tool for vascular dementia
c. It measures registration recall and long-term memory
d. On the three-step paper-folding task, the patient should be prompted at each step if he or she is unable to register it
e. The language part of the test covers a wide variety of frontal lobe functions

44) Regarding memory, all of the following statements are true, except:

a. Verbal short-term memory is stored in the left hemisphere
b. Visual short-term memory is stored in the right hemisphere
c. During encoding, the left side of the brain is activated
d. During retrieval, the right side of the brain is activated
e. Visuomotor knowledge is an aspect of the organization of short-term memory

45) Regarding memory, all of the following statements are true, except:

a. The visual association cortex is the anatomical correlate of iconic memory
b. The auditory association cortex is the anatomical correlate of echoic memory
c. The dominant parietal lobe is the anatomical correlate of auditory verbal short-term memory
d. The non-dominant temporo-occipital area is the anatomical correlate of visual verbal short-term memory
e. The non-dominant temporal lobe is the anatomical correlate of non-verbal short-term memory

46) Damage to which of the following brain structures results in an inability to store new memory?

a. Medial temporal lobes and hippocampus
b. Entorhinal cortex
c. Subiculum
d. Parahippocampal cortex
e. All of the above

47) All of the following statements about implicit memory are true, except:

a. It is recalled automatically without effort
b. It is learnt slowly through repetition
c. It is readily amenable to verbal reporting
d. Its storage requires functioning of the cerebellum
e. Classical and operant learning involve implicit memory

48) Regarding the language areas of the brain, all of the following statements are true, except:

a. Broca's area is involved in coordinating the organs of speech to produce coherent sounds
b. In lesions confined to Broca's area, the muscles involved in speech production are affected
c. Wernicke's area is involved in making sense of speech and language
d. Lesions of the angular gyrus produce an inability to read or write
e. Damage to the arcuate fasciculus results in a conduction dysphasia

49) Which of the following statements about agnosia is true?

a. Agnosia may result from impairment in the sensory pathways
b. Frontal lobe lesions usually cause pseudoagnosia
c. Lesions in the right occipital lobe result in apperceptive agnosia
d. Lesions in the left parieto-occipital areas result in associative agnosia
e. Astereognosia is the inability to recognize numbers or letters traced on the palm

50) Frontal lobe lesions can cause:

a. Pallilalia
b. Echolalia
c. Logoclonia
d. Motor Jacksonian fits
e. All of the above

1. Advanced psychological processes and treatments: Neuropsychology: Answers

1) a.

Prosopagnosia is a neuropsychological condition in which the patient is unable to recognize faces. 'The man who mistook his wife for a hat' is a well-known clinical story exemplifying this condition. The recognition of other environmental objects is preserved. There are radiological and pathological findings indicating the association of disconnection of the left inferior temporal cortex from the visual association area in the left parietal lobe leading to prosopagnosia. In a similar condition, associative visual agnosia results from bilateral medial occipitotemporal lesions, where the patient is also unable to name the objects but the ability to draw them is preserved. Both conditions occur in advanced Alzheimer's disease and with vascular pathology.

2) c.

Apperceptive agnosia patients are unable to identify and draw objects using visual cues. In this condition, other sensory modalities are preserved. It is thought to be a result of impaired transmission of information from the higher visual sensory pathway to visual association areas. Bilateral pathology in visual association areas is associated with the development of apperceptive agnosia. In a similar condition, associative visual agnosia patients are able to draw the item, but are unable to name it, as a result of medial occipital temporal lesions occurring bilaterally.

3) a.

The triad of Balint's syndrome includes optic ataxia (the inability to direct optically guided movements), oculomotor apraxia (the inability to direct the gaze rapidly) and simultanagnosia. Failure to acknowledge blindness is Anton's syndrome, which is seen with bilateral occipital lesions.

4) e.

Gerstmann's syndrome has been attributed to dominant parietal lobe lesions.

5) c.

Sound localization is mediated by the non-dominant hemisphere in the brain. Lexical processing (the extraction of vowels, consonants and words from the auditory input) is done in the higher language association areas in the left temporal lobe. Word deafness is intact hearing for voices but an inability to recognize speech, thought to be due to a disconnection of the auditory cortex from Wernicke's area.

6) e.

In limb-kinetic apraxia, the patient is unable to use the hand on the opposite side of the lesion (contralateral hand), although the strength of that hand is preserved. In ideomotor apraxia, the patient is not able to perform a motor act when the command is given. However, the patient is able to understand the command and the strength of muscles is preserved. Patients will also be able to perform the same act spontaneously. A lesion in Wernicke's area resulting in impairment in obeying verbal commands and a lesion in the left premotor area resulting in an impairment in the motor programming can cause ideomotor apraxia. In ideational apraxia, the patient is able to perform the individual components of a complex motor task, but unable to perform the entire act as a whole.

7) c.

In pure word deafness (verbal auditory agnosia), the defect is restricted to the understanding of spoken speech. In pure word blindness (alexia without agraphia), the difficulties are entirely restricted to understanding the written word. In pure word dumbness, the patient can comprehend both spoken speech and written material without difficulty; the defect is restricted to the production of spoken speech, which is marked by slurring and dysarthria, and the patient cannot speak at will, repeat words heard or read aloud.

8) d.

In Wernicke's dysphasia, the primary deficit is in the comprehension of spoken speech; speech is faulty but fluent and produced without effort.

9) d.

Broca's dysphasia is expressive dysphasia; writing is affected in parallel with speaking, and comprehension is relatively intact. Speech is characteristically sparse, slow and hesitant, with marked disturbances of rhythm, inflexion and articulation. Wrong words are often chosen and marked reiteration and perseveration are common. The patient usually recognizes his or her mistakes and attempts to correct them.

10) d.

The visual subtests in the Wechsler Adult Intelligence Scale include digit span.

11) e.

The level of word reading ability achieved by an adult has been shown to correlate highly with intelligence and, being well practised and overlearned, it proves to be relatively resistant to influences that impair other aspects of cognitive function. The National Adult Reading Test (NART) uses irregularly spelled words, which do not conform to rules (e.g. 'ache', 'bouquet', 'naive', etc.), and depends on correct pronunciation and strong familiarity. It is highly culture bound and is mainly used for patients with English as their first language.

12) a.

Raven's Progressive Matrices are used in clinical practice as a rapid device for estimating performance IQ. Usually the Mill Hill Vocabulary Test is also used to rapidly estimate verbal ability. The Bender-Gestalt Test is a rapid screening test of perception used to detect brain damage. The Visual Object and Space Perception Battery is another test for visual perception. The Behavioural Inattention Test is designed to examine unilateral visual neglect. The Token Test is sensitive to a minor degree of impairment of language comprehension.

13) b.

The Kendrick Object Learning Test is less stressful and more acceptable to elderly patients, and is used in the assessment of dementia. Patients with dominant temporal lobe damage show little impairment with the Ray−Osterrieth Test, which involves copying a complex geometrical design. On the revised version of the Wechler Memory Scale, practice effects cannot be avoided if testing is repeated, because the revision is presented in only one form. The shortened version of the Rivermead Behavioural Memory Test, used with aphasic patients, has been shown to be sensitive to the effects of memory deficits rather than language impairment.

14) d.

Tests of verbal fluency include the FAS Test. Patients with a left-sided frontal defect perform particularly badly on the Stroop Test.

15) e.

The Halstead−Reitan Battery also helps to determine whether the brain injury is located in the right or left hemisphere. It includes the Critical Flicker Frequency Test, the Tactual Performance Test, the Rhythm Test, the Speech Sound Perception Test, the Finger Tapping Test, the Time Sense Test, the Halstead−Wepman Aphasia Screening Test, and the Trait Making Test.

16) e.

DEMQOL is a new measure to assess health-related quality of life in people with dementia. It is a 28-item interviewer-administered questionnaire answered by the person with dementia. AGECAT is a computer program derived from the Geriatric Mental State Examination, which arrives at levels of confidence for diagnosing organic brain syndrome, schizophrenia, depression, etc.

17) b.

The Minnesota Multiphasic Personality Inventory emphasizes major psychopathology. The 16 Personality Factor Questionnaire is used in research in the non-clinical population. The Personality Assessment Inventory includes measures of psychopathology, personality dimensions, validity scales, and specific concerns to psychotherapy treatments. The Eysenck Personality Questionnaire is useful only as a screening device.

18) e.

Although used clinically, the greatest use for these scales is as research instruments; they help to standardize a subject cohort and provide objective outcome measures for assessing treatment response.

19) d.

Response sets are attitudes or styles in responding to personality questionnaires. Some people answer incorrectly to present themselves in a more favourable light to please the examiner. Others attempt to look worse than they truly are. Well-designed tests like the Minnesota Multiphasic Personality Inventory have built-in scales designed to detect such response sets and to adjust scores accordingly.

20) b.

Other clinical scales include the Hypochondriasis Scale, the Psychopathic Deviance Scale, the Paranoia Scale, the Psychasthenia Scale, the Schizophrenia Scale, and the Hypomania Scale.

21) c.

The Sentence Completion Test is brief in administration time, and can be useful in clinical interviews as an adjunct, if supplied beforehand.

22) d.

In anosognosia there is a lack of awareness of disease, particularly of hemiplegia, most often following a right parietal lesion.

23) e.

The Luria–Nebraska Neuropsychological Battery assess a wide range of cognitive functions, including memory, motor functions, tactile, auditory and visual functions, speech, and writing.

24) d.

Attitudes tend to predict behaviour best when they are (1) strong and consistent; (2) specifically related to the behaviour being predicted; (3) based on a person's direct experience; and (4) when the person is aware of his or her attitudes.

25) e.

The Sentence Completion Test is a subjective (projective) test. Other projective tests include the Rorschach Test, the Thematic Apperception Test, the Draw-a-Person Test and the Children's Apperception Test.

26) b.

The other three are logical-mathematical intelligence, spatial intelligence and interpersonal intelligence.

27) e.
The originator of factor analysis, Spearman (1904), proposed that individuals possess a general intelligence factor (g) and special factors (s) specific to particular abilities or tests. According to Spearman, factor g is the major determinant of performance on intelligence tests.

Spearman C. General intelligence, objectively determined and measured. *Am J Psychol* 2004; 15: 201–93.

28) e.
Social acceptability error describes the tendency to give answers expected by the interviewer.

29) d.
IQ is the ratio of mental age to chronological age $\times$ 100; it has a normal distribution, with a mean of 100 and a standard deviation of 15. Measured intelligence increases up to 16 years of age and plateaus until 25, after which it declines. Both the Stanford–Binet and the Wechsler scales are fairly valid predictors of achievement in school.

30) c.
Criterion validity refers to predictive validity and concurrent validity together. Incremental validity indicates whether the measurement being assessed is superior to other measurements in approaching true validity.

31) e.
The Present State Examination is one of the most reliable means of assessment of severe mental illness available for research. It has been used in important studies such as the International Pilot Study of Schizophrenia.

WHO. *Schizophrenia: An International Follow-Up Study*. Chichester: John Wiley & Sons, 1979.
Wing JK, Cooper JE, Sartorius N. *The Measurement and Classification of Psychiatric Symptoms*. Cambridge: Cambridge University Press, 1974.

32) e.
The Schedules for Clinical Assessment in Neuropsychiatry also allow DSM-IIIR diagnoses; a computer-assisted version is available.

33) d.
The International Personality Disorder Examination assesses phenomenology and life experiences, to enable psychiatric diagnosis according to ICD-10 and DSM-IIIR. It has 153 items and includes open-ended enquiries and questions to determine frequency, duration and age of onset.

34) e.
CATEGO is a computer program based on the Present State Examination (PSE) that gives a symptom score and a diagnosis.

35) a.
The Hamilton Anxiety Scale (HAS) was designed to be employed solely with anxiety disorders and not for rating anxiety in patients with other disorders.

36) e.
PANSS also rates social withdrawal and lack of spontaneity.

37) e.
There is also a version with symptom subscales for somatic symptoms, anxiety and insomnia, depression and social dysfunction.

38) c.
Wartenberg's reflex is a corneo-mandibular reflex and is considered to be primitive (when the corneal side of the lesion is touched, the mandible moves to the contralateral side). Witzelsucht is euphoria elaborated into a tendency to make jokes, puns or factitious remarks. Perseveration is performance of a particular action beyond its relevance. Magnetic syndrome is a type of behaviour in which a grasp reflex is coupled with an irrepressible tendency to follow objects with the hands when they are touched or when they enter the field of vision.

39) c.
In simultanagnosia there is usually no difficulty in forming other meaningful concepts, since auditory information is quickly understood. Anosognosia implies lack of understanding of disease.

40) c.
Hemiasomatognosia is the feeling that the limbs on one side are missing. Microsomatognosia is the feeling of abnormal smallness of body parts. Autoscopy is the hallucinatory perception of one's own body image projected into external visual space.

41) c.
In limb-kinetic apraxia, the skill and delicacy of movements are disturbed, but it is a function of muscular complexity rather than psychomotor complexity. In ideomotor apraxia, the patient can formulate an idea but is not able to execute it, though the instructions are understood. In ideational apraxia, the patient is unable to carry out coordinated sequences of actions, but is able to copy simple actions; this usually coexists with ideomotor apraxia.

42) e.
The Blessed Dementia Rating Scale is a measure of activities of daily living. The Hachinski Ischaemic Score helps differentiate between Alzheimer's dementia and vascular dementia. CAMCOG is the cognitive subscale of the CAMDEX.

Butler R, Pitt B (eds). *Seminars in Old Age Psychiatry*. London: Gaskell, 1998.

43) a.
The Mini Mental State Examination is used only as a screening tool in dementia assessment; it measures registration recall, but not long-term memory; the three-step paper-folding task should not be prompted at each step; the language part of the test covers only limited frontal tests, which is regarded as a drawback.

44) e.
Visuomotor knowledge and motor skills are aspects of the organization of long-term memory.

45) d.
The dominant temporo-occipital area is the anatomical correlate of visual verbal short-term memory.

46) e.
Explicit memory involves all these structures. Memory probably passes from medial temporal lobe structures after a few weeks or months to longer-term storage in the cortex.

47) c.
Implicit memory is not readily amenable to verbal reporting; storage requires functioning of the cerebellum and amygdala; specific sensory and motor systems are used in the learned task, e.g. the basal ganglia in motor skills.

48) b.
In lesions confined to Broca's area, the muscles involved in speech production work normally. Damage to the arcuate fasciculus results in a conduction dysphasia in which the person cannot repeat what is said to him or her. Comprehension and verbal fluency remain intact.

49) d.
Agnosia is the inability to interpret and recognize the significance of sensory information that does not result from impairment in the sensory pathways. Occipital lobe lesions cause pseudoagnosia. Lesions in the right parietal lobe result in apperceptive agnosia. Agraphaesthesia is the inability to recognize numbers or letters traced on the palm. Astereognosia is the inability to recognize objects by palpation.

50) e.
> Reiteration of phrases just spoken (echolalia), of single words (pallilalia) or a terminal syllable (logoclonia) are perseverative errors of speech occurring in frontal lobe damage.

Further reading

Butler R, Pitt B (eds). *Seminars in Old Age Psychiatry*. London: Gaskell, 1998.

Gelder M, Harrison P, Cowen P. *Shorter Oxford Textbook of Psychiatry*, 5th edn. Oxford: Oxford University Press, 2006.

Hodges JR. *Cognitive Assessment for Clinicians*, 2nd edn. Oxford: Oxford University Press, 2007.

Lishman WA. *Organic Psychiatry: The Psychological Consequences of Cerebral Disorder*, 3rd edn. Oxford: Wiley/Blackwell, 1997.

Puri B, Hall A. *Revision Notes in Psychiatry*, 2nd edn. London: Arnold/ Hodder Education, 2004.

Sadock BJ, Sadock VA. *Kaplan and Sadock's Synopsis of Psychiatry*, 10th edn. Baltimore, MD: Lippincott Williams and Wilkins, 2008.

2. Advanced psychological processes and treatments: Personality and personality disorder, developmental psychopathology (including temperament) and therapy models: Questions

1) In the New York Longitudinal Study (Thomas and Chess 1984):

   a. The most stable trait was 'approach or withdrawal to novelty', which seems the same thing as the extroversion–introversion polarity
   b. Most children (65%) could be categorized into three broad groupings: easy, difficult and slow to warm up
   c. Those exposed to parental conflict at age 3 were more likely to have poor adult social adjustment
   d. 'Poor fit' between a child's temperament and parental/teacher expectations was a risk factor for child maladjustment
   e. All of the above

2) Freud's concepts include all of the following, except:

   a. The unconscious mind must exist because people say and do more than they are 'aware of' or 'mean to'
   b. Every mental event is affected by previous ones
   c. The selective unconscious 'forgetting' of events too painful or objectionable to the conscious mind
   d. At some early stage the infant gets the idea of being fed from 'out there' (by the 'good breast'), but when the infant is hungry the 'out there' must be holding off (the 'bad breast')
   e. From birth into the second year, an infant has both libidinal and aggressive drives centred on 'oral eroticism', e.g. sucking, and 'oral sadism', e.g. biting

3) All of the following terms are associated with Freud, except:

   a. Transitional object
   b. Oedipal complex
   c. Electra complex
   d. Introjection
   e. Pleasure principle

4) Behavioural dimensions indicating inborn temperamental attributes include:

   a. Activity level
   b. Rhythmicity
   c. Approach or withdrawal
   d. Adaptability
   e. All of the above

5) Regarding attachment, which of the following statements is true?

a. Bonding is the same as attachment
b. Mary Ainsworth described attachment behaviour
c. John Bowlby described the sequential pattern of protest, despair and detachment as the infant's response to separation from the caretaker
d. Attachment behaviour starts at 6 months after birth
e. Inanimate objects cannot provide a secure base effect

6) Stranger anxiety:

a. Appears in the first month
b. Is more likely to occur in babies exposed to a variety of carers
c. Is identical to separation anxiety
d. Is fully established by 8 months
e. Does not occur when the infant is in the mother's arms

7) In learning theory, all of the following are true, except:

a. Drugs of abuse can act as a positive reinforcement at the biological level
b. Negative reinforcement can exacerbate the avoidance response in phobic avoidance states
c. In cognitive learning, more information leads to more effective and predictable outcomes
d. Extinction occurs as part of stimulus generalization
e. A prison sentence that follows long after the crime has been committed may not affect future criminal behaviour

8) Piaget's developmental stage corresponding to Freud's latency stage is the:

a. Sensorimotor stage
b. Formal operational stage
c. Preoperational stage
d. Concrete operational stage
e. Formal operations stage

9) In the management of psychosis, one of the benefits of psychodynamic understanding is that:

a. It helps to identify psychological stressors
b. It helps to identify personal significance in psychotic symptoms
c. It helps to clarify underlying vulnerability
d. It is useful in family meetings in which the aim is to understand the stresses and strains families face
e. All of the above

10) According to the psychoanalytic theory of depression:

   a. Mourning and depression are types of biopsychological reactions to loss
   b. The self undergoes an alteration through becoming identified with the lost object
   c. Hostility is turned inward
   d. The superego is coloured by the individual's own hostile and envious feelings
   e. All of the above

11) Which of the following is characteristic of attachment bonds?

   a. Attachment bonds are not persistent
   b. Attachment bonds involve a specific figure who is interchangeable
   c. The relationship within the dyad is emotionally not significant
   d. The individual wishes to maintain proximity to or contact with the attachment figure
   e. The individual does not feel distress at involuntary separation from the attachment figure

12) According to Freud's theory of personality development, all of the following statements are true, except:

   a. Excessive oral gratification or deprivation can result in libidinal fixations that lead to pathological traits like excessive optimism, narcissism, pessimism and demandingness
   b. Anal eroticism and fixation on its defences may create maladaptive character traits like orderliness, obstinacy, stubbornness and parsimony
   c. In the urethral stage, the main issues involve castration anxiety in males and penis envy in females
   d. Excess of inner control in the latency stage can lead to premature closure of personality development and precocious elaboration of obsessive character traits
   e. The genital stage involves partial reopening, reworking and reintegrating of all previous unsuccessful resolutions and fixations

13) Narcissistic defences include:

   a. Projection
   b. Introjection
   c. Regression
   d. Displacement
   e. Sublimation

14) Neurotic defences include:

   a. Intellectualization
   b. Rationalization
   c. Reaction formation
   d. Displacement
   e. All of the above

15) Mature defences include:

   a. Altruism
   b. Anticipation
   c. Asceticism
   d. Humour
   e. All of the above

16) In psychoanalytic theory, all of the following are true, except:

   a. Neurotic symptoms develop as a failure of repression
   b. It emphasizes the importance of superego formation in the construction of character
   c. Exaggerated development of certain character traits at the expense of others leads to personality disorders
   d. The expulsion of the drives or wishes from conscious awareness through repression or other defence mechanisms makes those drives less powerful and influential
   e. Traumatic events that seem to threaten survival may break through defences when the ego has been weakened

17) All of the following are true about Jung's personality theory, except:

   a. It rejects Freud's concept of the unconscious
   b. Archetypes are described as representational images and configurations with universal symbolic meanings
   c. Complexes develop as emotionally toned ideas
   d. A major developmental goal in adult life is individualization
   e. Anima refers to a man's undeveloped femininity and animus refers to a woman's undeveloped masculinity

18) All of the following statements are true about superego development in the psychoanalytic theory of personality development, except:

   a. Superego is developed through identification with parents
   b. Superego contains the individual's moral conscience
   c. Superego anxiety occurs after the resolution of the oedipal complex
   d. Superego develops before the child enters the oedipal stage
   e. The scrutiny activities of superego occur largely unconsciously

19) According to the stages of separation individualization proposed by Margaret Mahler, normal rapprochement includes all of the following, except:

a. It occurs between 18 and 24 months
b. Children realize their helplessness and dependence
c. The need for independence alternates with the need for closeness
d. Children move away from their mother and come back for reassurance
e. Children gradually comprehend and are readily reassured by the presence of their mother and other important people

20) Regarding temperament, which of the following statements is true?

a. The concept of parental fit does not take account of the temperamental characteristics of the child
b. Thomas and Chess used the term 'goodness to fit' to characterize the harmonious and consonant interaction between a mother and a child
c. According to Bates, temperament concepts cannot be defined as the patterns of surface behaviour
d. The neural basis of temperament is thought to emerge from the cerebellum
e. Characteristics of temperament in infants and preschool children do not predict adjustment in middle childhood and adolescence

21) In the preschool period:

a. Children do not understand that there may be more than one point of view to a moral issue
b. A problem may result if the needs of a newborn baby prevent the mother from attending to a first-born child's needs
c. By the age of 4, children are usually able to engage in cooperative play
d. Imaginary companions most often appear in the preschool years
e. All of the above

22) Regarding adoption, all of the following statements are true, except:

a. Adoptive parents most often tell their children of their status between the ages of 2 and 4 years
b. Emotional and behavioural disorders have been reported to be higher among adopted than non-adopted children
c. The later the age of adoption, the lower is the incidence and the less severe are any behavioural problems
d. An adopted child may split two sets of parents into good and bad parents
e. Forty per cent of adopted children are born to mothers aged between 15 and 19 years

23) Rutter's observations about parenting styles include all of the following, except:

    a. The authoritarian style leads to low self-esteem and social withdrawal in children

    b. The indulgent−permissive style leads to low self-reliance and aggression in children

    c. The indulgent−neglectful style leads to low self-esteem and aggression in children

    d. The authoritative−reciprocal style leads to low self-reliance and impaired self-control in children

    e. Firm rules and shared decision-making is the style most likely to result in self-reliance, self-esteem and a sense of social responsibility

24) In Erikson's stages of the life cycle, which of the following statements is true about the psychopathological outcomes associated with each stage if it is not mastered successfully?

    a. Basic mistrust is a major contribution to the development of schizoid personality disorder

    b. If shame and doubt dominate over autonomy, obsessive personality develops

    c. Excessive guilt between the ages of 3 and 5 years is associated with the development of schizophrenia

    d. In stage 4, development of inferiority can lead to severe work inhibitions and feelings of inadequacy in adult life

    e. Disorders during the stage of identity versus role diffusion include conduct disorder and psychotic disorders

25) Which of the following names is not paired with the correct term in the study of personality disorders?

    a. Rush−Moral derangement

    b. Pinel−Manie sans délire

    c. Kraepelin−Moral insanity

    d. Henderson−Psychopathic states

    e. Cleckley−Sociopathy

26) All of the following are true about personality theories, except:

    a. Eysenck's approach was categorical rather than dimensional

    b. Normothetic theories are based on studies of populations

    c. Ideographic theories relate to individual uniqueness

    d. Kelly's personal constructs, being unconscious, are formed at earlier developmental stages

    e. Bannister's Repertory Grid can be used to measure formal thought disorder

27) Regarding genetic and environmental factors that contribute to personality disorders, all of the following statements are true, except:

a. Among monozygotic twins the concordance for personality disorders is several times that among dizygotic twins
b. Research shows that there is a difference in concordance for personality disorders in monozygotic twins reared together and apart
c. Cluster A personality disorders are more common in the biological relatives of patients with schizophrenia
d. Depression is common in the family backgrounds of patients with borderline personality disorder
e. There is more association between schizotypal personality disorder and schizophrenia than with schizoid personality disorder and schizophrenia

28) Regarding biological factors that contribute to personality disorders, all of the following statements are true, except:

a. Persons who exhibit impulsive traits often show high levels of testosterone
b. Patients with obsessive compulsive personality disorders show shortened REM latency and abnormal results on dexamethasone suppression tests
c. College students with high platelet monoamine oxidase (MAO) levels spend more time in social activities than students with low platelet MAO levels
d. Smooth pursuit eye movements are saccadic in persons who are introverted
e. Slow-wave activity on EEG occurs in antisocial and borderline personality disorders

29) Regarding psychoanalytic factors of personality disorder, which of the following is true?

a. Freud suggested that personality traits are related to a fixation at one psychosexual stage of development
b. Wilhelm Reich coined the term 'character armor' to describe characteristic defensive styles
c. Persons with paranoid personality disorder use projection as their character armor
d. Persons with schizoid personality disorder use withdrawal as their character armor
e. All of the above

30) Understanding defence mechanisms in personality disorders is important, as exemplified in all of the following statements, except:

a. In schizoid personality disorder, recognition of the patient's fear of closeness and respect for his or her eccentric ways are therapeutic
b. In histrionic personality disorder, often therapists deal best with dissociation and denial by using displacement
c. The therapist should not allow obsessive compulsive personalities with characteristic isolation to control their own care
d. In therapy, projection is best dealt with by the agreement that therapists can disagree with patients' beliefs, rather than accepting that the beliefs may be true
e. Gently confronting a patient with the fact that no one is all good or bad is an effective way to deal with splitting

31) A 28-year-old woman inpatient with a diagnosis of borderline personality disorder cuts her wrists. Which is the most probable defence mechanism?

a. Acting out
b. Passive aggression
c. Displacement
d. Splitting
e. Reaction formation

32) All of the following are true about paranoid personality disorder, except:

a. Patients are affectively restricted and appear to be unemotional
b. It can be distinguished from borderline personality disorder because paranoid patients are rarely capable of overly involved, tumultuous relationships with others
c. Psychotherapy is the treatment of choice
d. If a therapist is accused of inconsistency or being at fault, honesty and apology are preferable to a defensive explanation
e. Paranoid patients usually do very well in group psychotherapy

33) All of the following statements are true about schizoid personality disorder, except:

a. Patients usually reveal a lifelong inability to express anger
b. Patients do not usually have a normal capacity to recognize reality
c. Onset usually occurs in early childhood
d. In psychotherapeutic settings, patients tend towards introspection
e. In group therapy, schizoid persons should be protected against aggressive attacks by group members for their proclivity to be silent

34) All of the following are true about schizotypal personality disorder, except:

    a. Ideas of reference, illusions and de-realization are part of a schizotypal person's everyday world

    b. If psychotic symptoms appear, they are brief and fragmentary

    c. Schizotype is regarded as the premorbid personality of the patient with schizophrenia

    d. A long-term study by McGlashan et al. reported that 25% of those with schizotypal personality disorder eventually commit suicide

    e. Magical thinking occurs in schizotypal personality disorder

35) Which of the following is true of antisocial personality disorder?

    a. It is classified as a type of personality disorder in ICD-10

    b. It is equally prevalent in men and in women

    c. Soft neurological signs occur, suggesting minimal brain damage in childhood

    d. Jails are more useful in alleviating the disorder than self-help groups

    e. The symptoms steadily increase up to the age of 35, with a peak of antisocial behaviour around the age of 30

36) All of the following are true in borderline personality disorder, except:

    a. Through a primitive defence mechanism of projective identification, intolerable aspects of the self are projected on to others

    b. The patient shows abnormal reasoning abilities on structured tests

    c. The patient shows deviant processes on unstructured projective tests

    d. Everybody is considered either all good or all bad

    e. It is twice as common in women as in men

37) Group psychotherapy with outpatients is usually not beneficial in people with:

    a. Alcohol dependence

    b. Schizophrenia

    c. Borderline personality disorder

    d. Depressive disorders

    e. Post-traumatic stress disorder

38) Regarding theories of personality development, all of the following are true, except:

a. According to Kelly's personal construct theory, anxiety results when the individual is presented with events outside his or her range of personal constructs
b. Bannister's Repertory Grid can be used to assess an individual's attitudes with respect to a series of bipolar constructs
c. Roger's self theory states that the most important aspect of personality is one's own view of oneself compared with the ideal self
d. According to Rotter's theory of locus of control, those attributing events to an external source are more confident about changing their life and environment
e. Kretschmer linked body build with personality

39) Regarding the outcome of the personality disorder, all of the following are true, except:

a. The aim of supportive psychotherapy in borderline personality disorder may be to diminish suicidal behaviour
b. Borderline personality disorder patients with high impulsiveness are most responsive to treatment
c. In antisocial personality disorder, there is an association between the patient's ability to form a relationship with the therapist and the treatment outcome
d. Borderline personality disorder tends to become less evident with age
e. Obsessive compulsive personality disorder does not tend to remit with age

40) All of the following are correctly paired, except:

a. Psychodrama–Moreno
b. Founder of analytical psychology–Freud
c. Transactional analysis–Berne
d. Self-psychology–Kohut
e. Psychobiology–Meyer

41) Interpersonal attraction is increased by:

a. Similarity
b. Proximity
c. Familiarity
d. Reciprocal self-disclosure
e. All of the above

42) Regarding social influence, all of the following statements are true, except:

  a. Task performance can be enhanced or diminished by the presence of others
  b. Complex or novel tasks or hostility from others can adversely affect performance
  c. Facilitation that occurs when others are simply observing is known as the audience effect
  d. A democratic leadership style leads to diminished productivity
  e. According to Deutsh and Gerard, informational conformity is evident with ambiguous stimuli

43) Conformity increases with:

  a. Group number
  b. Self-reliance
  c. Intelligence
  d. Expressiveness
  e. All of the above

44) Studies of small groups have shown all of the following, except:

  a. Group cohesiveness tends to be diminished when the group is competing with other groups
  b. The active involvement of participants in a discussion is not necessary for their level of arousal to change
  c. A group may take a riskier decision than its separate individuals would take
  d. They adopt an effective leadership style for the nature of the task
  e. The more rewarding the group, the more cohesive it is

45) Institutional rearing without an opportunity to form an attachment in infancy may result in all of the following, except:

  a. Shallow emotional relationships in later life
  b. Unselective attachment behaviour in later childhood
  c. Autism
  d. Developmental language delay
  e. Social deprivation

46) Which of the following statements about adolescence is true?

  a. Identity diffusion occurs in almost all teenagers
  b. If reached, the formal operational stage allows testing of different hypotheses
  c. Experiencing adolescent turmoil is important for future development
  d. Compared with childhood, family factors contribute more to the development of schizophrenia
  e. Adolescent girls are more sexually active than boys of the same age

47) Which of the following strategies are useful when dealing with dependence features in psychotherapy?

   a. Emphasize the time-limited nature of therapy from the outset
   b. Explicitly discuss the issue as part of the shared case conceptualization
   c. Encourage clients to attribute improvements to their own efforts
   d. End therapy gradually; establish together how the therapist can be replaced in the client's support system
   e. All of the above

48) All of the following statements are true about cognitive behavioural therapy, except:

   a. It was developed by Bion
   b. It encourages client–therapist collaboration
   c. It usually lasts several weeks
   d. It involves constructing a 'testable' conceptualization of the patient's problems
   e. It involves behavioural experiments aimed at cognitive change

49) Which of the following statements is true of secure attachment in mammals?

   a. It is involved in regulation of affects through modulation of the noradrenergic system
   b. It has a role in the development of the right orbitofrontal cortex
   c. It promotes exploratory behaviour and learning
   d. It is associated with successful social relationships with peers and successful parenting in adulthood
   e. All of the above

50) Regarding brief interventions for alcohol problems, all of the following statements are true, except:

   a. There is a correlation between duration of intervention and subsequent reduction in alcohol consumption
   b. They are effective in reducing attendance at A&E departments
   c. Stepped care is a model in which choice of the intervention is guided by the severity of the individual's alcohol problem
   d. Screening and brief intervention have a strong evidence base, with a recent Cochrane review showing efficacy in clinical practice
   e. There is no optimal duration for the treatment

2. Advanced psychological processes and treatments: Personality and personality disorder, developmental psychopathology (including temperament) and therapy models: Answers

1) e.
Children of 'difficult' temperament at age 3 (especially those exposed to parental conflict) were more likely to have poor adult social adjustment. 'Poor fit' can be reduced by counselling and education.

Thomas A, Chess S. Genesis and evolution of behavioral disorders: from infancy to early adult life. *Am J Psychiatry* 1984; **141**: 1–9.

2) d.
'Good breast/bad breast' is a concept proposed by Melanie Klein. That every mental event is affected by previous ones is psychic determinism. Forgetting events too painful or objectionable to the conscious mind is repression.

3) a.
The term 'transitional object' is associated with Donald Winnicott (1896–1971).

4) e.
Thomas and Chess identified nine behavioural dimensions. The others include intensity of reaction, threshold of responsiveness, quality of mood, attention span and persistence, and distractibility.

Thomas A, Chess S. *Temperament and Development.* New York: Brunner/Mazel, 1977.

5) c.
Bonding is the intense emotional and psychological relationship a mother develops with her baby. Attachment is the relationship the baby develops with its caregivers. Bowlby described attachment behaviour and Ainsworth developed it. Attachment behaviour starts from birth. Inanimate objects can provide a secure base effect; ones doing so were described by Winnicott as transitional objects.

6) d.
Stranger anxiety appears around 26 weeks, more commonly in babies exposed to a single carer. Separation anxiety occurs at between 10 and 18 weeks and is related to stranger anxiety but is not identical.

7) d.

Extinction is the gradual disappearance of a conditioned stimulus; generalization is the process whereby the same response is evoked by a similar stimulus.

8) d.

The concrete operational stage is between 7 and 11 years, when egocentric thought is replaced by operational thought and critical achievements are mastering the concepts of conservation and reversibility.

9) e.

Psychodynamic understanding also reveals the psychodynamic mechanisms operating in psychosis to avoid painful realities. It informs the phasing of recovery and suggests steps to tackle underlying vulnerability, thus contributing to relapse prevention.

10) e.

Emotional ambivalence deriving from early childhood relationships and losses is crucial.

11) d.

Attachment bonds are persistent; the specific figure is not interchangeable; the relationship within the dyad is emotionally significant; the individual feels distress at involuntary separation.

12) c.

In the urethral stage, the issues are urethral performance and loss of control; in the phallic stage, the main issues are castration anxiety in males and penis envy in females.

13) a.

Other narcissistic defences are denial and distortion; immature defences include acting out, blocking, hypochondriasis, introjection, passive aggressive behaviour, regression, schizoid fantasy and somatization.

14) e.

Other neurotic defences include controlling, externalization, inhibition, isolation, dissociation, repression and sexualization.

15) e.

Mature defences also include sublimation and suppression.

16) d.

The expulsion of the drives or wishes does not make them less powerful or influential; as a result, the unconscious tendencies fight their way back to consciousness (e.g. the disguised neurotic symptoms).

17) a.
Jung expanded Freud's concept of the unconscious by describing collective unconsciousness as consisting of all humankind's common, shared mythological and symbolic past. This includes archetypes and complexes.

18) d.
Superego is not formed until the oedipal complex is resolved and superego anxiety occurs around that time. The superego initially is the internalization of parental standards and values that include the ego ideal (what one should do) and moral conscience (what one should not do).

19) e.
Children gradually comprehend and are readily reassured by the presence of their mother and other important people in the stage of object constancy, at between 2 and 5 years.

20) b.
Parental fit takes account of the temperamental characteristics of both parent and child. According to Bates, temperament concepts can be defined at three levels: as patterns of surface behaviour, as a pattern of nervous system response and as having inborn genetic roots. The neural basis of temperament is thought to emerge from the limbic structures, the association cortex and the motor cortical areas. Characteristics of temperament in infants and preschool children predict adjustment in middle childhood and adolescence.

Bates J. Concepts and measures of temperament. In: Kohnstamm G, Bates J, Rothbart M (eds). *Temperament in Childhood*. Wiley: New York, 1989: 3–27.

21) e.
Children aged 3–6 are aware of their genitalia, and the differences between the sexes. Sibling rivalry appears, and growth can be traced through their drawings.

22) c.
The later the age of adoption, the higher is the incidence and the more severe are any behavioural problems.

23) d.
The authoritative–reciprocal style characterized by firm rules and shared decision-making is the style most likely to result in self-reliance, self-esteem and a sense of social responsibility.

24) c.
Excessive guilt in children aged between 3 and 5 years is associated with the development of generalized anxiety disorders and phobia. In stage 6,

persons with schizoid personality remain isolated; stage 7 features increased use of alcohol; stage 8 is characterized by a severe depressive episode.

25) c.
Kraepelin first defined the psychopathic personality and Prichard first described moral insanity.

26) a.
Using factor analysis, Eysenck identified the following personality traits: neuroticism/stability; extroversion/introversion; psychoticism/stability; intelligence.

27) b.
One study has shown that there is no difference in concordance for personality disorders in monozygotic twins reared together and apart.

Bergeman CS, Plomin R, McClearn GE, *et al*. Genotype–environment interaction in personality development: Identical twins reared apart. *Psychology Aging* 1988; **3**: 399–406.

28) c.
Low platelet MAO levels have been associated with activity and sociability in monkeys. College students with low platelet MAO levels spend more time in social activities than students with high platelet MAO levels. Low levels have also been noted in some patients with schizotypal disorders.

29) e.
Wilhelm Reich's theory has had a broad influence on contemporary concepts of personality disorders, as each person's unique personality is considered to be largely determined by his or her characteristic defence mechanisms.

30) c.
Whenever possible, the therapist should allow obsessive compulsive personalities with characteristic isolation to control their own care and should not engage in a battle of wills.

31) b.
Passive aggression is one of the characteristic defence mechanisms observed in people with personality disorders. Their anger and hostility are turned towards themselves, and self-destructive acts including deliberate self-harm may occur. Many clinicians agree that the best way to deal with such behaviour is to help patients express their feelings by ventilating their anger.

32) e.
Paranoid patients usually do not do very well in group psychotherapy, although it can be useful for improving social skills and diminishing suspiciousness through role playing.

33) b.
Although schizoid persons appear lost in daydreams, they have a normal capacity to recognize reality.

34) d.
McGlashan *et al.* reported that 10% of those with schizotypal personality disorder eventually commit suicide.

McGlashan TH, Grilo CM, Skodol AE, *et al.* The Collaborative Longitudinal Personality Disorders Study: Baseline axis I/II and II/II diagnostic co-occurrence. *Acta Psychiatr Scand* 2000; **102**: 256–64.

35) c.
Antisocial personality disorder is classified in DSM-IV and the equivalent in ICD-10 is dissocial personality disorder. Its prevalence is three times higher in men. When patients feel that they are among peers, their lack of motivation for change disappears and self-help groups are more useful. Antisocial behaviour peaks in late adolescence and there are reports that the symptoms decrease when patients grow old.

36) b.
Most therapists agree that patients show ordinary reasoning abilities on structured tests, such as the Wechsler Adult Intelligence Scale.

37) c.
In borderline personality disorder, group psychotherapy has traditionally been avoided because borderline patients are considered too demanding and disruptive.

38) d.
According to Rotter's theory of locus of control, those attributing events to an internal source are more confident about changing their life and environment.

39) b.
Borderline personality disorder patients with low impulsiveness are most responsive to treatment.

40) b.
Jung is regarded as the founder of analytical psychology.

41) e.
Interpersonal attraction is also increased by perceived competence.

42) d.
A democratic leadership style yields greater productivity.

43) a.
Self-reliant, intelligent, expressive, socially effective individuals are least vulnerable to group pressure.

44) a.
Group cohesiveness tends to be reinforced when the group is competing with other groups.

45) c.
Enuresis and aggression also occur.

46) b.
Formal operation occurs at between 12 and 14 years and a feature of it is the ability to think abstractly. Girls enter puberty 2 years earlier than boys; they may start dating earlier, but they are less sexually active than boys of the same age.

47) e.
All these strategies are routinely used in CBT. It is generally accepted that there is no role for transference and countertransference in CBT. Beck *et al.* (1979) described the importance of these processes in CBT. The term 'interpersonal process issues' has been used to describe the patient's reactions to the therapy and therapist, as well as the therapist's reactions to therapy and the patient in CBT (Safran & Segal 1996).

Beck AT, Rush AJ, Shaw BF, *et al. Cognitive Therapy of Depression.* Chichester: John Wiley & Sons, 1979.
Safran JD, Segal ZV. *Interpersonal Process in Cognitive Therapy.* Lanham, MD: Jason Aronson, 1996.

48) a.
Cognitive behavioural therapy was developed by Beck; Bion developed group therapy.

49) e.
The earliest attachment figure conceivably acts as a primary affect regulator, one that ameliorates and terminates the infant's distress, augments within reasonable limits its experience of happiness and pleasure, and offers predictable and replicable affect regulation.

50) a.
Brief interventions last between 5 and 60 minutes, consist of no more than five sessions and focus on providing counselling and education. A single contact lasting as little as 5–10 minutes can reduce an individual's risky drinking (Kaner *et al.* 2007).

Kaner EF, Beyer F, Dickinson HO, *et al.* Effectiveness of brief alcohol interventions in primary care populations. *Cochrane Database Syst Rev* 2007; **18**: CD004148.

Further reading

Gelder M, Harrison P, Cowen P. Chapters 7–15 and 17–23. In: *Shorter Oxford Textbook of Psychiatry*, 5th edn. Oxford: Oxford University Press, 2006.

Gross R. *Psychology: The Science of Mind and Behaviour*, 5th edn. London: Hodder Education, 2005.

Puri B, Hall A. *Revision Notes in Psychiatry*, 2nd edn. London: Arnold/ Hodder Education, 2004.

Sadock BJ, Sadock VA. *Kaplan and Sadock's Synopsis of Psychiatry*, 10th edn. Baltimore, MD: Lippincott Williams and Wilkins, 2008.

Smith EE, Bem DJ, Nolen-Hoeksema S. *Atkinson and Hilgard's Introduction to Psychology*, 14th edn. Florence, KY: Wadsworth Publishing Company, 2003.

3. Advanced psychology, pharmacology and treatments: Questions

1) Regarding common factors of psychotherapy, all of the following statements are correct, except:
   a. The therapeutic relationship is the most important of the common factors of psychotherapy
   b. Intense and rapid emotional release is called abreaction
   c. Empathetic listening and providing information are important components of all forms of psychotherapy
   d. In all forms of psychological treatment, reasons for the patient's condition should be provided indirectly through questions and interpretations
   e. All psychological treatments contain an element of suggestion

2) Which of the following statements is true of transference?
   a. It becomes increasingly strong as treatment progresses
   b. Patients usually transfer feelings and attitudes from their relationship with their parents to the therapist
   c. When transferred feelings are good, transference is said to be positive
   d. It may lead to behaviour such as threats of suicide
   e. All of the above

3) Regarding counselling, all of the following statements are true, except:
   a. In the client-centred approach, counsellors take a passive role
   b. Problem-solving counselling is a highly structured form of counselling
   c. In interpersonal counselling, the therapist encourages patients to consider alternative ways of coping with their difficulties
   d. In psychodynamic counselling, the patient's emotional reactions to the counsellor are considered as a source of information about problems in other relationships
   e. Evidence from clinical trials indicates that debriefing improves the outcome of survivors of disasters

4) In grief counselling:
   a. It is helpful to forewarn a bereaved person about unusual experiences such as feeling as if the dead person were present
   b. The bereaved person should not be encouraged to view the body
   c. Parents with a still-born baby should not be encouraged to name the dead baby
   d. Parents with a still-born baby should not be encouraged to keep photographs of the body to look at later if they wish
   e. If possible, the bereaved person should not be asked to put away the dead person's belongings

5) Which of the following statements is true in relation to psychological therapies for abnormal grief?

   a. Crisis intervention is not helpful
   b. Brief dynamic therapy is more effective than a mutual support group
   c. Group psychotherapy is significantly beneficial for bereaved spouses
   d. There is evidence that it is helpful to provide psychotherapy for all bereaved persons
   e. In a controlled evaluation, guided mourning produced modest benefit

6) Regarding psychological therapies for late effects of childhood sexual abuse, all of the following statements are true, except:

   a. Dynamic approaches focus on understanding the effects of the trauma on self-esteem and emotional expressions
   b. Cognitive behavioural approaches emphasize how the current patterns of thinking affect the present behaviour
   c. Group therapy is contraindicated
   d. Various therapy methods allow patients to set the pace at which they talk about the experience of being abused
   e. The therapist should take special care not to suggest memories of sexual abuse

7) Regarding recovered memories and false memories in relation to sexual abuse in childhood, which of the following is true?

   a. Many victims have partial amnesia for the most stressful parts of the experience
   b. Complete amnesia for repeated stressful events followed by their recall is frequent
   c. There is evidence that memories of single non-abusive childhood events can be implanted by suggestion in 50% of subjects
   d. Clinicians have reported that up to 80% of memories recovered in therapy are confirmed by other evidence
   e. Clinical reports suggest that about 75% of patients reporting childhood sexual abuse describe long periods in which they did not remember the abuse

8) Caplan's description of stages of coping include all of the following, except:

   a. Denial and disbelief
   b. Emotional arousal with efforts to solve the problem
   c. Greater arousal, leading to disorganization of behaviour
   d. Trials of alternative ways of coping
   e. Exhaustion and decompensation

9) Which of the following statements is true concerning supportive psychotherapy?

    a. Opportunity should be given for repeated release of emotions
    b. Reassurance should be offered in the first session
    c. It is sometimes appropriate for doctors to use their powers of persuasion to help patients to take some necessary steps
    d. Listening is not very important, as the therapy focuses more on information and advice
    e. It is useful to direct dependence to the therapist rather than directing it to a group of staff members caring for the patient

10) Several clinical trials have shown that interpersonal therapy is effective for:

    a. Depressive disorders in adults
    b. Depressive disorders in adolescents
    c. Dysthymia
    d. Bulimia nervosa
    e. All of the above

11) All of the following statements are true about interpersonal therapy, except:

    a. Treatment is carried out mostly in an unstructured way
    b. The initial assessment period lasts one to three sessions
    c. Among interpersonal problems, bereavement and other loss are considered
    d. To deal with role disputes and role transitions, patients are helped to negotiate with the other person
    e. Interpersonal deficits are discussed when analysing present relationship problems

12) All of the following statements are true about cognitive behavioural therapy, except:

    a. It is concerned with the ways the disorder developed in the past
    b. It focuses on the factors maintaining the disorder
    c. The patient takes an active part and the therapist is an expert advisor
    d. Therapeutic procedures are presented as experiments
    e. Treatment manuals ensure that different therapists use evidence-based procedures

13) Which of the following is a maintaining factor in the assessment for cognitive behavioural therapy?

    a. Avoidance
    b. Safety-seeking behaviours
    c. Selective attention
    d. The response of others
    e. All of the above

14) Regarding the maintaining factors identified in cognitive behavioural therapy, all of the following statements are true, except:

a. Avoidance prevents the extinction of the anxiety response
b. Escape from the anxiety-provoking situation is followed by a fall in anxiety, which reinforces the phobic avoidance
c. Children's unacceptable behaviour is reduced if parents pay more attention to the behaviour
d. Intrusive thoughts provoke an immediate emotional reaction, usually of anxiety or depression
e. Dysfunctional beliefs and attitudes determine the way in which situations are perceived and interpreted

15) Patients with social phobias attend more to the critical behaviour than to signs of approval. This is an example of:

a. Illogical thinking
b. Selective attention
c. Selective abstraction
d. All-or-nothing thinking
e. Personalization

16) In cognitive behavioural therapy, laddering is:

a. A special form of interviewing
b. Used to construct a hierarchy
c. The same as flooding
d. Used in modelling
e. Given as homework

17) In cognitive behavioural therapy, all of the following statements are true about the formulation, except:

a. The formulation is guided by the cognitive model of the disorder
b. An excessively critical parent is considered as a background factor in the disorder
c. A behaviour carried out because the person believes that it reduces an immediate threat but which in the long term perpetuates the person's concerns is described as an avoidance behaviour
d. A diagram on paper is used to build up the formulation step by step
e. The formulation is modified as necessary as a result of discussion with the patient

18) Regarding behavioural techniques, all of the following statements are true, except:

a. Relaxation training is useful for stress-related disorders like initial insomnia and mild hypertension
b. Exposure is used to reduce avoidance behaviour in phobic disorders
c. The results of flooding have been shown to be better than desensitization, as it is an intensive form of exposure
d. Exposure with response prevention is a treatment of obsessive compulsive disorder
e. Thought stopping is a distraction technique used to treat obsessive compulsive disorder

19) In exposure with response prevention, all of the following are true, except:

a. The therapist explains the rationale of the treatment
b. Patients may be faced with unexpected tasks
c. Modelling is used
d. Obsessional thoughts occurring without rituals are more difficult to treat
e. Habituation training is used

20) All of the following statements about contingency management are true, except:

a. It involves another person monitoring the behaviour
b. It includes identifying the stimuli and reinforcing them by recording events before and after the behaviour
c. It is never used alone in the treatment of substance abuse
d. It is used mainly in the treatment of people with learning disability
e. When applied to a group of patients living together, the arrangement is known as token economy

21) Regarding behavioural techniques, which of the following statements is true?

a. Social skill training is not useful in chronic mental disorder
b. An enuresis alarm is not very successful with children under the age of 6
c. Biofeedback may be of some value when normal sensory information is lost in spinal injuries
d. In aversion therapy, negative reinforcement is used to suppress unwanted behaviour
e. Habit reversal is a complex procedure used to treat Tourette's syndrome

22) Regarding the techniques used in cognitive restructuring, which of the following statements is true?

a. Thought stopping is a distraction technique
b. Neutralizing involves rehearsing a reassuring response
c. The therapist produces evidence that contradicts the beliefs
d. The patient's responsibility can be reassessed by constructing a pie chart
e. All of the above

23) Dialectic behavioural therapy:

a. Is delivered by a team of therapists and gives access by telephone to the therapist between sessions
b. Uses cognitive behavioural techniques, including self-monitoring
c. Uses the practice of detachment from experiences, known as mindfulness
d. Uses phrases that encapsulate the approach known as aphorisms
e. All of the above

24) In cognitive analytical therapy:

a. Traps are repetitive cycles of behaviour in which the consequences of the behaviour perpetuate it
b. Dilemmas are false choices or unduly narrow options
c. Snags are the anticipation of highly negative consequences of actions
d. Scaffolding is the provision of just enough support to enable patients to discover their own solutions
e. All of the above

25) All of the following are true about psychodynamic interpersonal therapy, except:

a. It uses the patient–therapist relationship as a tool for understanding and changing interpersonal problems
b. It uses more interpretation of transference than do other kinds of psychodynamic therapies
c. The therapist uses metaphor to communicate with patients
d. It has been tested in clinical trials in people who deliberately self-harm
e. It has been tested in clinical trials in people with Alzheimer's disease

26) Regarding special techniques used in couple therapy, all of the following statements are true, except:

a. Structural moves should not result in disagreement between partners
b. Reversed role-play is used to help the partners understand each other
c. In sculpting, partners take up positions, silently, to express some aspects of the relationship without words
d. Systemic tasks include making a timetable in which specific times are allocated for the interaction
e. Paradoxical injunctions are given as provocative statements designed to elicit a counter-response that the couple have previously resisted

27) All of the following are true about family therapy, except:
   a. It is used when young people living with their parents present with psychiatric problems
   b. It is often combined with antidepressant therapy in adults presenting with depression
   c. It is used in treating young people with anorexia after weight has been restored by other means, or who have a history of substance abuse or conduct disorder
   d. It is contraindicated in schizophrenia
   e. Circular questioning is often used to assess the family

28) Regarding treatment of personality disorders, all of the following statements are true, except:
   a. Psychological support is the mainstay of treatment, although medication should be considered as the first choice of treatment as it reduces hostility
   b. The atypical antipsychotics olanzapine and risperidone have been reported to reduce the hostility and chronic dysphoria of borderline personality disorder
   c. Fluoxetine is reported to be more effective than placebo in reducing anger in people with borderline personality disorder
   d. A randomized trial of valproate reported beneficial effects in borderline personality disorder
   e. Medications are generally better given to patients with borderline personality disorder than to those with dependence

29) All of the following statements are true about post-traumatic stress disorder (PTSD), except:
   a. Neurobiological studies suggest that hippocampal dysfunction prevents adequate memory processing
   b. Cognitive theories suggest that PTSD arises when the normal processing of emotionally charged information is overwhelmed and the memories persist in an unprocessed form
   c. Meta-analyses concluded that cognitive behavioural therapy is no more effective than inactive controls in terms of therapeutic effect size
   d. Treatment trials using eye-movement desensitization reprocessing have shown similar effect sizes to those obtained with cognitive behavioural therapy
   e. Meta-analysis carried out by the National Institute for Health and Clinical Excellence (NICE) indicated that drug treatment has a smaller effect size than structured psychotherapy

30) Regarding anxiety disorders, all of the following statements are true, except:

a. Cognitive behavioural therapy produces more improvement than no treatment in generalized anxiety disorder
b. The main treatment for specific phobia is SSRI antidepressants in the long term and benzodiazepines in the short term
c. Cognitive behavioural therapy is the psychological treatment of choice for social phobia, although SSRIs are often the first choice of treatment
d. Clinical trials indicate that, in the short term, cognitive therapy is about as effective as medication and in the long term it is probably more effective in agoraphobia
e. It was found that the combination of cognitive therapy and imipramine was no more effective in panic disorder than either treatment alone

31) Which of the following statements is true regarding obsessive compulsive disorder?

a. When given in high dose, clomipramine is more effective than placebo in reducing obsessional symptoms
b. There is some evidence to indicate that SSRIs are less effective than clomipramine
c. Exposure and response prevention result in substantial improvement in two-thirds of patients with moderately severe rituals
d. The immediate results of neurosurgery in severe cases are often a striking reduction in tension and distress
e. All of the above

32) Regarding conversion disorder, all of the following statements are true, except:

a. Social factors appear to be major determinants of the onset and development of conversion symptoms
b. Some of the phenomena classified as conversion disorders in Western countries may in some other cultures be accepted as possession disorders
c. For acute conversion disorders seen in primary care or hospital emergency departments, reassurance and suggestion of improvement are appropriate
d. Antidepressants and cognitive behavioural therapy were found to be very effective in long-term management
e. Patients who do not improve should be reviewed thoroughly for undiscovered physical illness

33) Which of the following statements is true about the use of tricyclic antidepressants in the acute treatment of depression?

a. They are clearly more effective than placebo in all but the most severely depressed patients
b. They are more effective in patients with depressive psychosis
c. They are more effective in milder depressive states (i.e. those with Hamilton depression scores of less than about 14)
d. They are more effective with atypical depression
e. All of the above

34) Regarding the treatment of depression, all of the following statements are true, except:

a. There is good evidence that cognitive behavioural therapy is more effective than a waiting-list control condition
b. A review by the National Institute for Health and Clinical Excellence (NICE) suggested that the combination of cognitive behaviour therapy with antidepressant medication was more effective than medication alone
c. There is sufficient evidence that cognitive behavioural therapy is more effective than other psychotherapies
d. SSRIs are more effective than tricylics where depression occurs in association with obsessive compulsive disorder
e. Venlafaxine is little more effective than SSRIs in patients with more severe depressive states

35) Assessment for cognitive behavioural therapy in obsessive compulsive disorder requires all of the following, except:

a. Knowledge of the degree of family involvement
b. Knowledge of the patient's degree of insight or overvalued ideation
c. Assessment of the patient's readiness to change
d. Analysis of countertransference
e. Assessment of the patient's reasons for holding beliefs

36) Placebo-controlled studies of the role of continuation therapy in unipolar depression have reached the conclusion that:

a. Continuing antidepressant treatment for 6 months past the point of remission halves the relapse rate
b. Treatment should be at the originally effective dose if possible
c. In a working age population at low risk of relapse, continuation of antidepressant treatment for longer than 6 months confers little benefit
d. In elderly people at low risk of relapse, continuation of antidepressant treatment for 12 months is more appropriate
e. All of the above

37) Regarding the treatment of recurrent mood disorders, all of the following statements are true, except:

a. Longer-term antidepressant maintenance treatment in recurrent depressive disorder reduces the relapse rate
b. The use of lithium in patients with recurrent mood disorders is associated with a significant reduction in mortality from suicide
c. Evidence supports the longer-term use of valproate in the maintenance treatment of bipolar disorder as it is more effective than lithium
d. Lamotrigine has a modest benefit in the prevention of mania and has a clearer prophylactic effect against depression
e. In the longer-term maintenance treatment of bipolar disorder, there is evidence that olanzapine is equivalent to lithium in overall efficacy

38) Regarding the treatment of mood disorders, which of the following statements is true?

a. Cognitive therapy in the acute stage of depression lessens the risk of subsequent relapse
b. There is research evidence that education about the early signs of relapse reduces the rate of manic illness in bipolar patients
c. Research in elderly depressed patients found that a combination of nortriptyline and interpersonal therapy was more effective than nortriptyline and clinical management in preventing depressive relapse over 3 years
d. The National Institute for Health and Clinical Excellence (NICE) recommends combining cognitive behaviour therapy and antidepressants in severe depression
e. All of the above

39) Effective psychosocial interventions for schizophrenia include:

a. Family therapy and psycho-education
b. Cognitive remediation
c. Social skills training
d. Assertive community treatment
e. All of the above

40) Regarding the treatment of schizophrenia, all of the following statements are true, except:

a. Drug treatment has most effect on the positive symptoms
b. Many controlled trials have shown the effectiveness of continued antipsychotic therapy
c. Depot medications are more successful than continued oral medication in preventing relapse
d. In clozapine-resistant schizophrenia, there is strong evidence in favour of augmentation with lamotrigine or valproate
e. Family interventions with education have been shown to lower the rates of hospitalization and improve medication compliance

41) Which of the following is true of premature ejaculation?

a. It is more common in older men
b. It can be treated with the start–stop technique
c. It can be treated with the squeeze technique
d. It can be treated with the quiet-vagina technique
e. SSRIs can be useful in its treatment

42) Regarding sexual dysfunction in men, all of the following statements are true, except:

a. Primary cases of erectile disorder may occur through a low sexual drive and anxiety about sexual performance
b. Erectile dysfunction and premature ejaculation are the most common sexual problems in men
c. Lack of sexual interest is the most common sexual problem in women
d. In sensate focus therapy, patients are strongly encouraged to check their own state of sexual arousal
e. Early studies suggested that sex therapy is successful in a third of patients

43) Regarding the prognosis of obsessive compulsive disorder, all of the following statements are true, except:

a. Two-thirds of cases improve to some extent within a year
b. Prognosis is better when there is a precipitating event
c. Prognosis is better when the symptoms are episodic
d. Prognosis is better when the onset is in childhood
e. Prognosis is worse when there is a personality disorder

44) Contraindications of brief insight-oriented therapy include:

a. Obsessional disorders
b. Hypochondriachal disorder
c. Severe mood disorder
d. Schizophrenia with past emotional problems causing present distress
e. All of the above

45) Electroconvulsive therapy causes all of the following, except:

a. Increased cerebral noradrenergic activity
b. Increased cerebral serotoninergic function
c. Increased cerebral tyrosine hydroxylase activity
d. Increased cerebral dopamine concentration
e. Increased cerebral acetylcholine concentration

46) All of the following statements about electroconvulsive therapy are true, except:

   a. It is a rapid and effective treatment for depressive stupor
   b. It may cause worsening of mania
   c. It is useful in the treatment of acute catatonic states
   d. It is effective for positive symptoms such as delusions and thought disorder in schizophrenia
   e. It was found to be useful in people with intractable Parkinson's disease

47) When is there an increased suicidal risk in schizophrenia?

   a. When there are frequent exacerbations of psychosis
   b. When there is good premorbid functioning
   c. Early in the course of the disorder
   d. During hospitalization or shortly after discharge
   e. All of the above

48) The psychological variables that may be associated with suicidal behaviour include:

   a. Dichotomous thinking
   b. Cognitive constriction
   c. Problem-solving deficits
   d. Overgeneralized autographical memory
   e. All of the above

49) All of the following are recommended in the care of suicidal patients in hospital, except:

   a. On admission, remove objects that might be used for suicide
   b. Do not discuss the care plans with the patient as it may make suicidal attempts easier
   c. Agree a visitor policy, including number of visitors, duration of visit and what they need to know
   d. Agree a date of discharge and plan aftercare in advance
   e. At discharge, prescribe in adequate but non-dangerous amounts

50) Components of motivational interviewing include:

   a. Expressing empathy
   b. Detecting and rolling with resistance
   c. Pointing out discrepancies in the history
   d. Raising awareness about the contrast between substance users' aims and behaviour
   e. All of the above

3. Advanced psychology, pharmacology and treatments: Answers

1) d.

The reasons for the patient's condition may be stated directly by the therapist, as in short-term therapy, or indirectly through questions and interpretations, as in long-term therapy. With the exception of hypnosis, suggestion is not deliberately increased in psychological treatments; however, all psychological treatments contain an element of suggestion.

2) e.

If transference is interpreted and addressed appropriately early on, it may be helpful for patients to understand the true origins of their feelings and behaviour not only for the therapist but more widely.

3) e.

Evidence from clinical trials indicates that debriefing does not improve the outcome of survivors of disasters, and methods using cognitive techniques may be more helpful.

4) a.

Grief counselling helps the person to accept that the loss is real, to work through the stages of grief and to adjust to life without the deceased. The bereaved person's viewing of the body or putting away the dead person's belongings, or the parents of a still-born baby being encouraged to keep photographs of the body to look at later if they wish, helps this transition.

5) e.

There is some evidence that crisis intervention may be helpful for people at high risk of an abnormal grief reaction (Raphael 1977); brief dynamic therapy is no more effective than a mutual support group (Marmar et al. 1988); group psychotherapy is no more effective than no treatment in bereaved spouses (Lieberman & Yalom 1992); in a controlled evaluation, guided mourning produced modest benefit (Clark 2004; Foa & Rothbaum 1997).

Clark A. Working with grieving adults. *Adv Psychiatr Treat* 2004; **10**: 164–70.

Foa E, Rothbaum B. *Treating the Trauma of Rape: Cognitive-Behavioral Therapy for PTSD*. New York: Guilford Press, 1997.

Lieberman MA, Yalom I. Brief group psychotherapy for the spousally bereaved: a controlled study. *Int J Group Psychother* 1992; **42**: 117–32.

Marmar CR, Horowitz MJ, Weiss DS, *et al*. A controlled trial of brief psychotherapy and mutual-help group treatment of conjugal bereavement. *Am J Psychiatry* 1988; **145**: 203–9.

Raphael B. Preventive intervention with the recently bereaved. *Arch Gen Psychiatry* 1977; **34**: 1450–4.

6) c.

The late effects of childhood sexual abuse have been treated with counselling, dynamic psychotherapy, cognitive therapy and group therapy.

7) a.

Complete amnesia for repeated stressful events followed by their recall is less frequent and for many clinicians improbable. There is evidence that memories of single non-abusive childhood events can be implanted by suggestion in 25% of subjects (Brewin 2007; McNally 2003). Clinicians have reported that up to 40% of memories recovered in therapy are confirmed by other evidence. Some 25–50% of people reporting childhood sexual abuse describe long periods in which they did not remember the abuse.

Brewin CR. Autobiographical memory for trauma: update on four controversies. *Memory* 2007; **15**: 227–48.
McNally RJ. Progress and controversy in the study of posttraumatic stress disorder. *Annu Rev Psychol* 2003; **54**: 229–52.

8) a.

Denial and disbelief are the first stage of grief; **b** to **e** are the four stages of coping described by Caplan. Crisis intervention seeks to limit the reaction to the first stage or, if it has been passed before the person seeks help, to avoid the fourth stage.

Caplan G. *Principles of Preventive Psychiatry*. New York: Basic Books, 1964.

9) c.

Supportive psychotherapy should not be attempted before using more active forms of psychotherapeutic interventions. Emotional release can be helpful in the early stages but repeated release is unlikely to be beneficial. Encouraging hope is important, but reassurance should be offered only when the patient's concerns have been fully understood. The therapeutic relationship, listening, information and advice, emotional release, encouraging hope and persuasion are important components of supportive psychotherapy.

10) e.

Interpersonal therapy was shown to be effective in depressive disorders in adults and adolescents by Mufson *et al.* (2004) and in dysthymia by Markowitz (2003).

Markowitz JC. Interpersonal psychotherapy for chronic depression. *J Clin Psychol* 2003; **59**: 847–58.
Mufson L, Dorta KP, Wickramaratne P, Nomura Y, Olfson M, Weissman MM. A randomized effectiveness trial of interpersonal psychotherapy for depressed adolescents. *Arch Gen Psychiatry* 2004; **61**: 577–84.

11) a.
Treatment is highly structured and the content of treatment and sessions is planned carefully.

12) a.
Cognitive behavioural therapy is not concerned with how the disorder has developed in the past, but focuses on the factors maintaining the disorder at the time of treatment. Behaviour therapy focuses on the factors that provoke the symptoms or abnormal behaviour. Cognitive therapy generally focuses on two kinds of abnormal thinking: intrusive thoughts and dysfunctional beliefs.

13) e.
One of the most frequent maintaining factors is avoidance (phobic and anxiety disorders). Many behaviours are maintained by their consequences (the response of others); increased attention is another reinforcer of behaviour. Two kinds of abnormal thinking that act as maintaining factors include intrusive thoughts and dysfunctional beliefs and attitudes. Three factors are thought to maintain dysfunctional beliefs and attitudes: attending selectively, thinking illogically and safety-seeking behaviour.

14) c.
Increased attention is a powerful reinforcer and children's unacceptable behaviour can be increased if parents pay more attention to the behaviour.

15) b.
Selective attention is attending selectively to evidence that confirms dysfunctional beliefs and attitudes, and ignoring or discounting evidence that contradicts them. Examples of illogical thinking include overgeneralization, selective abstraction, personalization and all-or-none thinking.

16) a.
Laddering is a special interviewing technique for use with patients who need help to become aware of and describe maladaptive beliefs. A series of questions is asked, each about the answer to the previous question.

17) c.
A behaviour carried out because the person believes that it reduces an immediate threat but in the long term perpetuates that person's concerns is described as safety-seeking behaviour, which is a maintaining factor.

18) c.
In flooding, patients enter the top of the hierarchy from the start. Many patients find it distressing and the results of flooding have not been shown to be more effective than desensitization; flooding is rarely used.

19) b.

Every task is agreed in advance and patients will never be faced with an unexpected task. Habituation training is a form of mental exposure treatment.

20) c.

Contingency management is used alone or as a part of a wider programme in the treatment of substance abuse.

21) b.

An enuresis alarm is not very successful in children under the age of 6, children who are uncooperative or children with associated psychiatric disorders.

22) e.

These principles are used in cognitive restructuring in the treatment of anxiety disorders, depression, eating disorders and psychosis.

23) e.

Dialectic behavioural therapy was developed by Marsha M. Linehan as a treatment for patients with borderline personality disorder. Treatment is highly structured and intensive, with individual sessions, skills training in a group and access to the therapist by phone, and lasts up to one year.

24) e.

Cognitive analytical therapy was developed by Anthony Ryle; the theory of reciprocal roles was developed when it was applied to borderline personality disorder. According to Ryle, people's internalized templates can be abnormal in three ways: (1) the repertoire of different roles is restricted; (2) roles cannot be switched easily; and (3) roles are inflexible.

25) b.

Psychodynamic interpersonal therapy was developed by Hobson. It uses less interpretation of transference than do other kinds of psychodynamic therapies, and has been tested in clinical trials in high utilizers of psychiatric services (Guthrie *et al.* 1999), chronic functional dyspepsia (Hamilton *et al.* 2000), deliberate self-harm (Guthrie *et al.* 2001) and Alzheimer's disease (Burns *et al.* 2005).

Burns A, Guthrie E, Marino-Francis F, *et al.* Brief psychotherapy in Alzheimer's disease: randomized controlled trial. *Br J Psychiatry* 2005; **187**: 143–7.

Guthrie E, Moorey J, Margison F, *et al.* Cost-effectiveness of brief psychodynamic-interpersonal therapy in high utilizers of psychiatric services. *Arch Gen Psychiatry* 1999; **56**: 519–26.

Guthrie E, Kapur N, Mackway-Jones K, *et al.* Randomized controlled trial of brief psychological intervention after deliberate self-poisoning. *BMJ* 2001; **323**: 135–8.

Hamilton J, Guthrie E, Creed F, *et al.* A randomized controlled trial of psychotherapy in patients with chronic functional dyspepsia. *Gastroenterology* 2000; **119**: 661–9.

26) a.
Structural moves include requiring disagreement, reversed role-play and sculpting. Couples may be asked to disagree about something when one partner dominates the other, who habitually gives in to avoid disagreement.

27) d.
Special kinds of family treatment have been developed to reduce relapses in schizophrenia.

28) a.
Medication should not be the first choice and when it is prescribed it should be part of a wider plan covering psychological and social needs (Tyrer & Bateman 2004).

Tyrer P, Bateman AW. Drug treatment for personality disorders. *Adv Psychiatr Treat* 2004; **10**: 389–98.

29) c.
A meta-analysis (Bradley et al. 2005) suggested that CBT has a therapeutic effect size of 1.65 compared with inactive controls. The neurobiological studies also suggest that increased activity in noradrenergic innervation of the amygdala increases arousal and facilitates the automatic encoding and recall of traumatic memories (O'Donnell et al. 2004).

Bradley R, Greene J, Russ E, *et al*. A multidimensional meta-analysis of psychotherapy for PTSD. *Am J Psychiatry* 2005; **162**: 214–27.
O'Donnell T, Coupland N, Hegadoren KM. Noradrenergic mechanisms in the pathophysiology of PTSD. *Neuropsychobiology* 2004; **50**: 273–83.

30) b.
The main treatment for specific phobia is the exposure form of behavioural therapy. Some patients seek help shortly before an important engagement made difficult by the phobia and then a few doses of benzodiazepines are prescribed. For other choices see Barlow et al. (1997), van Vliet et al. (1994) and Clark et al. (2003).

Barlow DH, Esler JL, Vitali AE. Psychosocial treatments for panic disorders, phobias, and generalized anxiety disorder. In: Nathan PE, Gorman JM (eds), *A Guide to Treatments That Work*. New York: Oxford University Press, 1997: 288–318.
Clark DM, Ehlers A, McManus F, *et al*. Cognitive therapy versus fluoxetine in generalized social phobia: a randomized placebo-controlled trial. *J Consult Clin Psychol* 2003; **71**: 1058–67.
van Vliet IM, den Boer JA, Westenberg HG. Psychopharmacological treatment of social phobia: a double blind placebo controlled study with fluvoxamine. *Psychopharmacology (Berl)* 1994; **115**: 128–34.

31) e.
Exposure and response prevention seems to produce better long-term results but it is difficult to achieve response prevention when symptoms are severe. Because of this, medication and response prevention are often combined.

32) d.
Medication has no direct role in the treatment, unless the disorder is secondary to depressive or anxiety disorders. Cognitive behavioural therapy appears to be of little specific value, though it may act as a non-specific aid to recovery.

33) a.
Tricyclics appear to be less effective in patients with depressive psychosis, milder depressive states (i.e. with Hamilton depression scores of less than about 14) and atypical depression.

34) c.
There is insufficient evidence that cognitive behavioural therapy is more effective than other psychotherapies. Neither is there sufficient evidence to show that cognitive behavioural therapy is more effective than placebo medication with clinical management or general practitioner treatment as usual.

35) d.
Analysis of countertransference is carried out only in dynamic therapies.

36) e.
About a third of patients withdrawn from medication relapse over the next year, with the majority of relapses occurring in the first 6 months (Anderson 2000, 2003).

Anderson IM. Selective serotonin reuptake inhibitors versus tricyclic antidepressants: a meta-analysis of efficacy and tolerability. *J Affect Disord* 2000; 58: 19–36.
Anderson IM. Drug treatment of depression: reflections on the evidence. *Adv Psychiatr Treat* 2003; 9: 11–20.

37) c.
At present, evidence supporting the longer-term use of valproate in the maintenance treatment of bipolar disorder is slender and less than that for lithium.

38) e.
Cognitive therapy in the acute stage of depression lessens the risk of subsequent relapse (Hollon *et al.* 2005). In a randomized controlled trial there was evidence that education about the early signs of relapse reduced the rates of manic illness in bipolar patients over 18 months by 30% (Perry *et al.* 1999).

Hollon SD, DeRubeis RJ, Shelton RC, *et al*. Prevention of relapse following cognitive therapy vs medications in moderate to severe depression. *Arch Gen Psychiatry* 2005; **62**: 417–22.

Perry A, Tarrier N, Morriss R, *et al*. Randomized controlled trial of efficacy of teaching patients with bipolar disorder to identify early symptoms of relapse and obtain treatment. *BMJ* 1999; **318**: 149–53.

39) e.

Cognitive behavioural therapy, supported employment, illness management skills and integrated treatment for comorbid substance abuse are other recognized psychosocial interventions.

40) d.

In clozapine-resistant schizophrenia, there is only weak evidence in favour of augmentation with lamotrigine or valproate; also, as a common augmentation strategy, a D2-receptor antagonist such as amisulpride or risperidone is used.

41) a.

Premature ejaculation is more common in younger men, especially during their first sexual relationships.

42) d.

Sensate focus therapy, described by Masters and Johnson, involves behavioural psychotherapy with graded assignments; patients are strongly discouraged from checking their own state of sexual arousal because this has an inhibiting effect.

43) d.

The prognosis is worse when onset is in childhood and when social and occupational adjustment is poor.

44) e.

Brief insight-oriented therapy is also contraindicated in some personality disorders that lead to acting out.

45) e.

Electroconvulsive therapy causes decreased cerebral acetylcholine concentration and increased cerebral acetylcholinesterase activity.

46) b.

Electroconvulsive therapy can lead to a rapid resolution of mania but is generally reserved for patients who do not respond to drug treatment or for those whose manic illness is severe.

47) e.

In addition to the demographic risk factors associated with suicide in other psychiatric disorders, such as male gender, social isolation, unemployment, and previous suicidal behaviour, these are factors specific to schizophrenia.

48) e.

All these could act by predisposing people to act impulsively (Williams & Pollock 2000).

Williams JMG, Pollock LR. The psychology of suicidal behaviour. In: Hawton K, van Heeringen K (eds), *International Handbook of Suicide and Attempted Suicide*, pp. 79–93. Chichester: John Wiley, 2000.

49) b.

Discussing and agreeing plans with the patient is recommended.

50) e.

Motivational interviewing is used in alcohol misuse. This interview style, which avoids arguing and is not judgemental, can help to persuade the patient to engage in a useful review of his or her current pattern of drinking.

Further reading

Gelder M, Harrison P, Cowen P. Chapters 21 and 22. In: *Shorter Oxford Textbook of Psychiatry*, 5th edn. Oxford: Oxford University Press, 2006.

Puri B, Hall A. *Revision Notes in Psychiatry*, 2nd edn. London: Arnold/ Hodder Education, 2004.

Sadock BJ, Sadock VA. *Kaplan and Sadock's Synopsis of Psychiatry*, 10th edn. Baltimore, MD: Lippincott Williams and Wilkins, 2008.

Taylor D, Paton C, Kerwin R. *Maudsley Prescribing Guidelines*, 9th edn. London: Informa Healthcare, 2007.

4. Neurosciences: Questions

1) Which of the following statements is true of MDMA?

   a. It stands for methamphetamine
   b. It has a street name of ecstasy
   c. It causes miosis and bradycardia
   d. Hypothermia and hypernatraemia are common complications of overdosage
   e. All of the above

2) Regarding Brodmann's areas, which of the following statements is false?

   a. Area 4 is the primary motor cortex
   b. Area 18 is the primary visual cortex
   c. Area 6 is the premotor cortex
   d. Area 44 and 45 form part of Broca's area
   e. Area 40 forms part of Wernicke's area

3) Which type of cell is found only in the cerebellum?

   a. Purkinje cell
   b. Granule cell
   c. Mossy fibre
   d. Pyramidal neurons
   e. Stellate cell

4) Action potential is produced when:

   a. Sodium ions move into the nerve cell
   b. Potassium ions move into the nerve cell
   c. Calcium moves into the nerve cell
   d. Calcium moves out of the nerve cell
   e. Sodium moves out of the nerve cell

5) The typical resting potential of a nerve cell is:

   a. -10 mV
   b. 80 mV
   c. -70 mV
   d. 100 mV
   e. -50 mV

6) A construction worker who had a recent fall has been referred by the medics for psychiatric consultation because of a change in behaviour. He has been inappropriate to ward staff and has been irritable but has not been seen to have any cognitive problems. He has lost interest in personal cleanliness. The most probable site of his lesion is:

a. Subcortical
b. Temporal
c. Parietal
d. Frontal
e. Occipital

7) Which of the following features can differentiate dementia from delirium?

a. Hallucinations
b. Altered sleep–wake cycle
c. Clear consciousness
d. Inappropriate behaviour
e. Disorientation

8) All of the following are levels of consciousnesss, except:

a. Alertness
b. Obtundation
c. Stupor
d. Coma
e. Paralysis

9) Regarding the Glasgow Coma Scale, which of the following statements is false?

a. The maximum score for verbal response is 5
b. The total score is 15
c. The patient scores 5 if able to localize pain in the best motor response subset
d. The patient scores 4 if able to open eyes to command in the eye-opening subset
e. The patient scores 1 if not able to respond verbally at all in best verbal response

10) The Digit-Repetition Test is used to assess:

a. Attention
b. Concentration
c. Memory
d. Activities of daily living
e. Language

11) Components of basal ganglia include:

a. Corpus striatum
b. Globus pallidus
c. Claustrum
d. Amygdaloid complex
e. All of the above

12) Which of the following does not describe the speech in Broca's aphasia?

a. Non-fluent
b. Dysarthric
c. Effortful
d. Agrammatic
e. Well articulated

13) All the following structures are involved in the storage and retrieval of verbal and non-verbal memory, except:

a. Hippocampus
b. Mammillary body
c. Red nucleus
d. Limbic structures
e. Dorsomedial nuclei of the thalamus

14) Which of the following statements is true of astereognosis?

a. It is usually due to a lesion in the posterior parietal lobe
b. It occurs only if there is a bilateral lesion
c. It is usually tested by asking the person to keep his or her eyes open and identify a common object in the hand
d. It is difficult to detect in persons with a primary sensory defect of the hand
e. It is a symptom of Gerstmann's syndrome

15) The Trail-Making Test is completed poorly by persons with a lesion in which of the following lobes?

a. Frontal
b. Temporal
c. Occipital
d. Parietal
e. Cerebellar

16) Which of the following is false regarding the WAIS-R (the Revised Wechsler Adult Intelligence Scale)?

   a. It can be used in clients between the ages of 16 and 74
   b. It has six subsets in the verbal scale
   c. It has six subsets in the performance scale
   d. It has subsets for both vocabulary and arithmetic in the verbal scale
   e. The verbal scale includes a subset for comprehension

17) Which of the following is not a usual symptom of the dominant lobe lesion?

   a. Aphasia
   b. Agraphia
   c. Anosognosia
   d. Alexia
   e. Dyscalculia

18) Biceps jerk involves which nerve segment?

   a. T3
   b. C3
   c. C6
   d. C7
   e. C5

19) Which peripheral nerve is involved in supinator jerk?

   a. Radial
   b. Deep branch of the ulnar nerve
   c. Musculocutaneous
   d. Median nerve
   e. Superficial branch of the ulnar nerve

20) The segmental innervations for knee jerk are:

   a. C5–T1
   b. L3–L4
   c. L4–L5
   d. T1
   e. T1–T2

21) Which of the following is true of Parkinsonian tremor?

   a. It is present at rest
   b. Its usual frequency is 1–4 Hz
   c. It is present even in voluntary movement with the affected body part
   d. It is caused by a lesion in the hypothalamus
   e. It is present during sleep

22) The eleventh cranial nerve can be tested by:

    a. Vocal cord examination
    b. Testing gag reflex
    c. Asking the patient to shrug the shoulders
    d. Rinne's test
    e. Weber's test

23) Which of the following statements is true regarding Foster Kennedy syndrome?

    a. It is caused by a tumour in the posterior inferior frontal region
    b. It may cause optic atrophy on one side
    c. It may lead to papilloedema on one side
    d. It may cause raised intracranial pressure
    e. All of the above

24) Which of the following statements is false regarding Balint's syndrome?

    a. It causes optic ataxia
    b. It causes oculomotor apraxia
    c. It causes simultanagnosia
    d. It is caused by frontal lesions
    e. It is caused by temporal lobe lesions

25) All of the following are part of the auditory pathway, except:

    a. Cochlear nerve
    b. Cochlear nuclei
    c. Inferior colliculus
    d. Lateral lemniscus
    e. Lateral geniculate body

26) The basal ganglia consist of all of the following, except:

    a. Corpus striatum
    b. Substantia nigra
    c. Thalamus
    d. Globus pallidus
    e. Caudate nucleus

27) Which of the following statements is false?

    a. Subthalamic nucleus lesion yields ballistic movements
    b. Reduced activity of the striatum leads to bradykinesia
    c. The caudate nucleus is shrunken in Huntington's disease
    d. The globus pallidus may be severely damaged in Wilson's disease
    e. The globus pallidus receives input from the corpus striatum

28) The limbic system consists of all of the following, except:

a. Mammillary body
b. Cingulate gyrus
c. Amygdala
d. Putamen
e. Orbitofrontal cortex

29) Which of the following statements is false?

a. Huntington's disease usually produces atrophy of the caudate nucleus
b. An MRI scan in vascular dementia shows patches of decreased signal in white matter
c. Neurosyphilis may produce a characteristic enhancement of the meninges, especially at the base of the brain
d. Multiple sclerosis plaques are easily seen on MRI scans as periventricular patches of increased signal intensity
e. The ventricles are dilated in normal-pressure hydrocephalus

30) In neurotransmission at the synapses, all of the following mediate the fusion of the vesicle to the inner surface of the presynaptic membrane, except:

a. Synaptophysin
b. Synaptotagmin
c. Synaptobrevin
d. Neurexins
e. Syntaxins

31) Which of the following statements is false regarding MRI studies?

a. The two parameters that are varied are the duration of the radiofrequency excitation pulse and the length of time that data are collected from the realigning nuclei
b. T1 MRI scans are most useful for assessing overall brain structure
c. Areas within brain tissue that have high water content appear dark on T2 images
d. Units of magnetic strength are rated in units of tesla
e. T2 images reveal brain pathology more clearly than T1

32) Features of upper motor neuron lesion include all of the following, except:

a. Extensor plantar response
b. Muscle wasting
c. Brisk tendon reflexes
d. Increased muscle tone
e. Muscle weakness

33) Which of the following is a feature of lower motor neuron lesion?

   a. Increased muscle tone
   b. Increased muscle mass
   c. Increased tendon reflexes
   d. Increased fasciculations
   e. Increased muscle strength

34) Which of the following sensations could be affected in the upper extremities in syringomyelia?

   a. Temperature
   b. Touch
   c. Vibration
   d. Proprioception
   e. Pressure

35) All of the following statements are true regarding the posterior column, except:

   a. Vibration sensations are lost in lesions of the column
   b. Romberg's sign is positive when the posterior column is affected
   c. It consists of fasciculus gracilis and fasciculus cuneatus
   d. There may be problems with proprioception when it is affected
   e. Temperature sensation is usually affected when it is damaged

36) Regarding Brown-Séquard syndrome, all of the following statements are true, except:

   a. It is caused by hemisection of the spinal cord
   b. It may be produced by inflammatory disease of the spinal cord
   c. It is characterized by ipsilateral dorsal column sensory loss
   d. Pyramidal signs usually occur on the contralateral side
   e. It is characterized by contralateral spinothalamic sensory impairment

37) Which of the following statements is true of Pott's disease of the spine?

   a. It is caused by osteoporosis of the spine
   b. Its first symptom is usually back pain
   c. It usually occurs in the lumbar vertebrae
   d. Treatment is by decompression only
   e. Collapse of vertebrae occurs early in the disease

38) Which of the following statements is false regarding Arnold–Chiari malformation?

   a. Cerebellar tonsillar herniation occurs in type I
   b. The cerebellum and lower part of the brain stem are herniated in type 2
   c. It is often associated with syringomyelia
   d. Symptoms usually present in childhood
   e. Treatment is foramen magnum decompression and shunting

39) Which of the following statements is false?

   a. Tropical spastic paraparesis is a slowly progressive disease caused by HTLV-I infection
   b. Optic atrophy is present occasionally in tropical spastic paraparesis
   c. Cystic dilatation of the third ventricle occurs in Dandy–Walker syndrome
   d. Use of sodium valproate during pregnancy can lead to spina bifida
   e. The lateral and posterior columns of the spinal cord are affected in subacute combined degeneration of the spinal cord

40) Which of the following statements is true of Klippel–Feil deformity?

   a. It is caused by fusion of the thoracic vertebrae
   b. It is associated with nerve deafness
   c. It may present with signs and symptoms of syringomyelia
   d. People with Klippel–Feil deformity usually have a long neck
   e. All of the above

41) Which of the following statements is false regarding motor neuron disease?

   a. There is degeneration of the anterior horn cells in the spinal cord
   b. There is no intellectual impairment in most patients
   c. The sensory tracts remain normal
   d. The motor neurons to the bladder and bowel sphincters are affected
   e. Progressive foot drop is a common presentation

42) Mononeuritis multiplex can be caused by:

   a. Diabetes
   b. Systemic lupus erythematosus
   c. Sarcoidosis
   d. Leprosy
   e. All of the above

43) Which of the following pairings of muscles with their corresponding nerve supply is false?

   a. Abductor pollicis brevis–Ulnar nerve
   b. Opponens pollicis–Median nerve
   c. Flexor carpi ulnaris–Ulnar nerve
   d. Brachioradialis–Radial nerve
   e. Supinator–Radial nerve

44) All of the following lead to polyneuropathy, except:

   a. Mumps
   b. Diabetes
   c. Guillain–Barré syndrome
   d. Trauma
   e. Vitamin B12 deficiency

45) In Guillain–Barré syndrome:

    a. The first symptoms are usually motor
    b. The cranial nerves are usually spared
    c. Bladder dysfunction is rare
    d. Cerebrospinal fluid pressure is high
    e. Cerebrospinal fluid shows a raised cell count of $10-200$ cells/mm^3

46) Which of the following statements is false regarding multiple sclerosis?

    a. It is rare in childhood
    b. It is uncommon over the age of 50
    c. Acute optic neuritis is mostly unilateral
    d. The lower motor neurons are commonly affected
    e. Erectile impotence and ejaculatory failure are common symptoms

47) Diffuse cerebral anoxia can be caused by:

    a. Cardiac arrest
    b. Fat embolism
    c. Cerebral malaria
    d. Cardiopulmonary bypass surgery
    e. All of the above

48) Which of the following statements is false regarding Wernicke–Korsakoff syndrome?

    a. Clinical features include the triad of ophthalmoplegia, ataxia and confusion
    b. It occurs only in alcoholics
    c. Hypothermia may occur because of hypothalamic involvement
    d. The third and fourth nerves may be affected
    e. Peripheral neuropathy may occur in most cases

49) Which of the following can cause ataxia?

    a. Phenytoin
    b. Carbamazepine
    c. Benzodiazepine
    d. Alcohol
    e. All of the above

50) Regarding benign intracranial hypertension, all of the following statements are true, except:

    a. There is a strong association with obesity
    b. Hypervitaminosis A in children may lead to benign intracranial hypertension
    c. It most commonly affects men over the age of 50 years
    d. Cerebrospinal fluid pressure may be more than $200-250$ mmHg
    e. A CT scan is usually normal or shows small ventricles

4. Neurosciences: Answers

1) b.
MDMA stands for 3,4-methylenedioxy-*N*-methylamphetamine. It causes mydriasis and tachycardia. Overdosage leads to hyperthermia and hyponatraemia, which should be managed urgently to prevent fatality. MDMA is a common subject in the examination.

2) b.
Area 17 is the primary visual cortex, while area 18 is the secondary visual cortex. The brain is divided into areas according to the cytoarchitecture, called Brodmann's areas.

3) a.
The Purkinje cells are large cells seen only in the cerebellum.

4) a.
The movement of sodium ions into the nerve cell activates the action potential.

5) c.
Resting membrane potential is always negative. Nerve cells maintain a resting membrane potential of around -70 mV.

6) d.
The features that have been described are typical of frontal lobe problems.

7) c.
One of the characteristic features differentiating dementia and delirium is that a demented patient will have clear consciousness while consciousness is altered in a patient with delirium.

8) e.
Paralysis is loss of muscle function. A completely paralysed person can still be alert and may respond with eye contact or eye movement. Obtundation refers to a transitional stage between stupor and lethargy.

9) d.
The Glasgow Coma Scale is a neurological scale used to rate the level of consciousness. It has three sections. In the eye response section, a score of 4 is given if eyes are opened spontaneously. The score is only 3 if eyes open to command.

10) a.
The Digit-Repetition Test assesses the attention of the person. A normal person can repeat five to seven digits without difficulty.

11) e.
Corpus striatum is comprised of caudate nucleus and putamen.

12) e.
Well-articulated speech is usually a feature of Wernicke's aphasia. All the others are characteristic of Broca's aphasia.

13) c.
The red nucleus is involved in motor coordination.

14) d.
Astereognosis is caused by a lesion in the anterior part of the parietal lobe. It is usually tested with the person's eyes closed.

15) a.
The Trail-Making Test is included in the Halstead–Reitan Battery.

16) c.
The verbal scale has six subsets: information, comprehension, arithmetic, similarities, digit span and vocabulary. The performance scale has only five subsets: picture completion, block design, picture arrangement, object assembly and digit symbol.

17) c.
Anosognosia is mostly caused by a lesion on the non-dominant side of the brain.

18) e.
The C5 nerve is tested by biceps jerk.

19) a.
The radial nerve needs to be intact for supinator jerk.

20) b.
Knee jerk is caused by L3–L4 innervation.

21) a.
Resting tremor is classically present and disappears when that part of the body is used.

22) c.

Normal shrugging of the shoulders elicits an intact eleventh nerve.

23) e.

Foster Kennedy syndrome is caused by a tumour in the posterior inferior frontal region.

24) e.

Balint's syndrome is due to bilateral parieto-occipital lesions. It leads to optic ataxia (inability to direct optically guided movements), oculomotor apraxia (inability to direct gaze rapidly) and simultanagnosia (inability to integrate a visual scene to perceive it as a whole).

25) e.

The lateral geniculate body is part of the visual pathway while the medial geniculate body is part of the auditory pathway.

26) c.

Sometimes the examination asks questions about the basic parts in neuroanatomy. A common question is on the basal ganglia, which consist of corpus striatum, globus pallidus, substantia nigra and subthalamic nuclei.

27) b.

Overactivity of the striatum leads to bradykinesia. This is due to lack of dopaminergic inhibition.

28) d.

The putamen is part of the basal ganglia.

29) b.

Vascular dementia is characterized by multiple infarcts in the brain. This is seen as increased signal in white matter.

30) a.

Synaptophysin helps to create a pore in the presynaptic membrane.

Sadock BJ, Sadock VA. Neurophysiology and neurochemistry. In: *Kaplan and Sadock's Synopsis of Psychiatry*, 10th edn. Baltimore, MD: Lippincott Williams and Wilkins, 2008.

31) c.

Areas within the brain tissue that have higher water content (for example because of inflammation or a tumour) appear brighter on T2-weighted images.

32) b.

Muscle wasting is usually seen with lower motor neuron lesions. With upper motor lesions there may be muscle weakness but no muscle wasting.

33) d.

Lower motor neuron lesions cause decreased muscle tone, flaccid paralysis and reduced tone. They lead to fasciculations.

34) a.

Syringomyelia is a condition whereby a cavity appears in the central canal for a variety of reasons. Classically it spares the dorsal column, leaving touch, vibration, proprioception and pressure unaffected.

35) e.

Temperature sensation is carried up the anterolateral column and hence would not usually be affected by posterior column lesions.

36) d.

Pyramidal signs usually occur on the ipsilateral side. If they occur bilaterally, they are commonly worse on the ipsilateral side.

37) b.

Pott's disease is due to tuberculosis of the spine. It usually affects the thoracic vertebrae of children and young adults. Treatment is by anti-tuberculosis chemotherapy. Decompression may be needed. Collapse of vertebrae occurs late.

38) d.

Arnold–Chiari malformation usually presents in adulthood.

Souhami R, Moxham J. Chapter 26. In: *Textbook of Medicine*, 4th edn. London: Churchill Livingstone, 2002.

39) c.

Cystic dilatation of the fourth ventricle occurs in Dandy–Walker syndrome.

40) c.

Klippel–Feil deformity is due to fusion of the cervical vertebrae. People with the deformity have a short neck and a low posterior hair-line, and they may have associated conduction deafness. There may be an association with syringomyelia.

41) d.

One of the differentiating features from other neurological conditions is that the motor neurons to the bladder and bowel nerve sphincters are spared.

42) e.
Mononeuritis multiplex or multifocal neuropathy can be due to all the listed diseases. For details of other causes refer to Souhami & Moxham (2002).

Souhami R, Moxham J. Chapter 26. In: *Textbook of Medicine*, 4th edn. London: Churchill Livingstone, 2002.

43) a.
Abductor pollicis brevis is part of the thenar muscles and is supplied by the median nerve.

44) d.
Trauma causes mononeuropathy or multiple mononeuropathy rather than polyneuropathy.

45) c.
In Guillain–Barré syndrome, the first symptoms are usually sensory. Cranial nerve involvement occurs in 30–40% of patients. Cerebrospinal fluid pressure is usually normal and the fluid shows a normal cell count.

46) d.
The lower motor neurons are rarely affected in multiple sclerosis.

47) e.
All of these can lead to diffuse cerebral anoxia.

48) b.
Wernicke–Korsakoff syndrome is due to thiamine deficiency and can occur in other conditions, such as starvation and severe malnutrition.

49) e.
All of these can cause ataxia.

50) c.
Benign intracranial hypertension most commonly affects young women.

Further reading

Gelder M, Harrison P, Cowen P. Chapters 21 and 22. In: *Shorter Oxford Textbook of Psychiatry*, 5th edn. Oxford: Oxford University Press, 2006.

Guyton C, Hall JE. *Textbook of Medical Physiology*, 11th edn. London: Saunders, 2005.

Kasper DL, Braunwald E, Hauser A, Fauci AS, Longo D, Jameson JL. *Harrison's Principles of Internal Medicine*. New York: McGraw-Hill, 2005.

Kumar P, Clarke M. *Clinical Medicine*, 6th edn. London: Saunders, 2005.
Sadock BJ, Sadock VA. *Kaplan and Sadock's Synopsis of Psychiatry*, 10th edn. Baltimore, MD: Lippincott Williams and Wilkins, 2008.
Snell RS. *Clinical Neuroanatomy for Medical Students*, 5th edn. Baltimore, MD: Lippincott Williams & Wilkins, 2001.

5. Genetics and basic neurosciences: Questions

1) A patient asks you about a recent newspaper report on the neuregulin-1 gene and psychiatric disorder. You explain to her that the most likely psychiatric link is with which one of the following disorders?

   a. Anorexia nervosa
   b. Attention deficit hyperactivity disorder (ADHD)
   c. Bulimia nervosa
   d. Major depressive disorder
   e. Schizophrenia

2) Transfer of information from the DNA molecule to the primary RNA is called:

   a. Translation
   b. Transcription
   c. Inheritance
   d. Mosaicism
   e. Linkage

3) Regarding autosomal-dominant inheritance, which of the following statements is false?

   a. The phenotypic trait is present in all individuals carrying the dominant allele
   b. Male-to-male transmission can take place
   c. Disorder is transmitted only if both parents are homozygous
   d. Vertical transmission can take place
   e. Males and females can be affected

4) In X-linked recessive inheritance, all of the following statements can be true, except:

   a. Female heterozygotes are carriers
   b. Male-to-male transmission can occur
   c. Males with the abnormal allele manifest the phenotypic trait
   d. Both the X chromosomes need to have the abnormal allele in a female for the trait to be manifested
   e. The X-linked recessive traits are rarer than the X-linked dominant traits

5) Which of the following is not a technique used in molecular genetics?

a. Cutting
b. Splicing
c. Grinding
d. Blotting
e. Recombination

6) All of the following disorders are due to trisomy, except:

a. Down syndrome
b. Edwards syndrome
c. Patau syndrome
d. Cri-du-chat syndrome
e. Trisomy 23

7) All of the following are X-linked dominant disorders, except:

a. Aicardi syndrome
b. Rett syndrome
c. Marfan syndrome
d. Vitamin D resistant rickets
e. Fragile X syndrome

8) The likelihood of a person with a particular genotype presenting with the associated phenotype is called:

a. Concordance
b. Probands
c. Penetrance
d. Index case
e. Susceptibility

9) All of the following are X-linked recessive disorders, except:

a. Cerebellar ataxia
b. Hurler syndrome
c. Lesch–Nyhan syndrome
d. Lowe syndrome
e. Duchenne muscular dystrophy

10) The prevalence rate of Alzheimer's dementia over the age of 95 is:

a. 15%
b. 82%
c. 43%
d. 50%
e. 67%

11) If concordance for a psychiatric disorder is higher in monozygotic twins than in dizygotic twins, a genetic component is presumed; the greater the difference in concordance, the greater the ...:
   a. Heritability
   b. Sensitivity
   c. Penetrance
   d. Ambiguity
   e. Number of people affected

12) Which of the following statements is false regarding genetic studies of personality disorders?
   a. Heritability of antisocial behaviour is seen more in adults
   b. Shared environmental factors are more important in the aetiology of antisocial behaviour in children and adolescents than in adults
   c. Adoptees separated at birth from persistent antisocial parents have higher rates of antisocial personality behaviour than do adoptees whose parents are not antisocial
   d. Antisocial personality disorder is diagnosed more often in men than women
   e. Biological parents of children who are not antisocial show more antisocial behaviour than do the biological parents of antisocial children

13) A nitrogenous base (e.g. adenine) and sugar (e.g. ribose or deoxyribose) give rise to:
   a. A nucleotide
   b. DNA
   c. mRNA
   d. tRNA
   e. A nucleoside

14) Which of the following statements is true regarding DNA replication?
   a. Synthesis can occur only in the 5'−3' direction
   b. DNA replication ends at a replication fork
   c. Hydrogen bond holding the two DNA strands are cut by ligase
   d. Polymerase helps in binding the Okazaki fragments
   e. Uracil is used instead of thymine in DNA

15) Regarding DNA synthesis, all of the following statements are true, except:
   a. Synthesis on the leading strand is by DNA polymerase δ
   b. Synthesis on the lagging strand is by DNA polymerase α
   c. Okazaki fragments are synthesized from the leading strand
   d. Synthesis of DNA is called semi-discontinuous
   e. Synthesis of DNA is called semi-conservative

16) Genetic studies include which of the following:

a. Recombinant fraction
b. Restriction endonuclease
c. Southern blotting
d. Twin studies
e. All of the above

17) Which of the following statements is true regarding autosomal abnormalities?

a. Most cases of Down syndrome are due to translocation of genetic material between chromosome 21 and another
b. Edwards syndrome relates to trisomy 13
c. Prader–Willi syndrome is due to partial deletion of the short arm of chromosome 15
d. Cri-du-chat syndrome is due to deletion on the short arm of chromosome 5
e. Deletion on chromosome 13 can lead to Wilms' tumour

18) All of the following statements are true regarding men with Klinefelter syndrome, except:

a. They are often infertile
b. They usually present with gynaecomastia
c. The phenotypic male has an extra Y chromosome
d. They may have a disproportionate body shape
e. Their IQ is often normal

19) Which of the following statements is false regarding females with Turner syndrome?

a. They usually have long stature
b. They can be diagnosed by buccal mucosa cell chromosomal analysis
c. They have an XO genotype
d. They usually have associated cardiovascular defects
e. Craniofacial abnormalities include micrognathia, low-set ears and downward-slanting palpebral fissures

20) Which of the following statements is false regarding fragile X syndrome?

a. It is also called Martin–Bell–Renpenning syndrome
b. Most people with the syndrome have normal IQ
c. Speech is usually high pitched and often nasal
d. People with the syndrome have short stature
e. Males with the syndrome present with macro-orchidism

21) Which of the following is an autosomal-dominant syndrome with characteristic features of tall stature, long slim limbs and arachnodactyly?

    a. Caplan syndrome
    b. Down syndrome
    c. Edwards syndrome
    d. Turner syndrome
    e. Marfan syndrome

22) Which of the following statements is true?

    a. Capping and polyadenylation are types of post-translational processing
    b. Transcription proceeds in the $3'-5'$ direction
    c. The anti-codon is seen on the tRNA
    d. AUG is also known as the termination codon
    e. Transcription follows translation in gene expression

23) All of the following statements are true regarding Duchenne muscular dystrophy, except:

    a. It is an X-linked recessive disease
    b. It is mainly seen in females
    c. Symptoms are usually manifested before the age of 6 years
    d. The disorder is caused by a mutation in the DMD gene
    e. In affected individuals, creatine phosphokinase-MM levels in the bloodstream are extremely high

24) 'Artificial embryo twinning' and 'somatic cell nuclear transfer' are procedures specifically related to:

    a. Gene therapy
    b. Stem cell therapy
    c. Cloning
    d. DNA extraction
    e. None of the above

25) What are the missing words? RNA contains base ... in place of base ... in DNA.

    a. Uracil–Guanine
    b. Uracil–Thymine
    c. Adenine–Guanine
    d. Adenine–Thymine
    e. None of the above

26) Which of the following statements is false regarding Smith–Lemli–Opitz syndrome (SLOS)?

    a. It is a metabolic disorder caused by a mutation on chromosome 11
    b. The disease mainly pertains to hampered synthesis of an enzyme responsible for cholesterol synthesis
    c. SLOS is inherited in an autosomal-dominant pattern
    d. Cleft palate and polydactyly are symptoms related to SLOS
    e. People with SLOS usually present with mental retardation

27) Which of the following statements is false regarding phenylketonuria (PKU)?

    a. Individuals affected always have a normal IQ
    b. PKU is due to a mutation on chromosome 12
    c. The main pathology is due to excess phenylalanine
    d. PKU can be detected by high-performance liquid chromatography (HPLC) or the Guthrie test
    e. It is inherited as an autosomal-recessive disease

28) Classical galactosaemia affects one in every how many newborn infants?

    a. 10 000
    b. 55 000
    c. 135 000
    d. 500
    e. None of the above

29) People with cystic fibrosis inherit a defective gene called CFTR (cystic fibrosis transmembrane conductance regulator) on which chromosome?

    a. Chromosome 14
    b. Chromosome 11
    c. Short arm of chromosome 3
    d. Chromosome 5
    e. Chromosome 7

30) Which of the following is true about alpha-1-antitrypsin deficiency?

    a. It is a common genetic cause of liver disease in children
    b. It usually manifests in the fifth decade
    c. It is easily differentiated from other respiratory abnormalities like emphysema, asthma, etc.
    d. It affects only the lungs
    e. Alpha-1-antitrypsin is synthesized mainly in the lungs

31) Which of the following has the lowest heritability estimate?

a. Schizophrenia
b. Bipolar disorder
c. Alcohol problem or dependence
d. Major depression
e. Generalized anxiety disorder

32) Regarding genetic variations, all of the following statements are true, except:

a. Polymorphisms or allelic variants occur on average every 1000 nucleotides across the whole genome
b. Most polymorphisms involve a change in a single nucleotide
c. Most polymorphisms are clinically significant with functional correlates
d. In linkage studies, a LOD score of more than 3 is conventionally taken as reasonable evidence for linkage
e. All chromosomes can be studied in genome wide linkage scans

33) Regarding genetic polymorphisms in psychiatry, which of the following statements is true?

a. The APOE4 variant gene on chromosome 19 is identified as a risk factor for Alzheimer's disease
b. COMT Val158Met polymorphism is identified as a risk factor for schizophrenia
c. COMT Val158Met polymorphism may predict response to antipsychotic drugs
d. 5-HT transporter gene polymorphism predisposes to depression following early life events
e. All of the above

34) The Papez circuit includes:

a. The hippocampus
b. The fornix
c. The mammillary bodies
d. The anterior nucleus of the thalamus
e. All of the above

35) Regarding neuronal migration, all the following statements are true, except:

a. It mainly occurs in the first 6 months of gestation
b. It is guided by radially oriented astrocytic glial fibres
c. Heterotopic neurons within the frontal lobe and failure to complete axonal path finding are thought to be associated with pathology in schizophrenia
d. The peak of synaptogenesis occurs in gestation
e. In normal development the subplate neurons degenerate

36) Which of the following is a criterion for a neurotransmitter?

 a. It is synthesized in the neuron
 b. It is present in the presynaptic neuron and is released on depolariz-
 ation in physiologically significant amounts
 c. When administered exogenously as a drug, it should mimic the effects
 of the endogenous neurotransmitter
 d. A mechanism in the neurons or synaptic cleft acts to remove or
 deactivate it
 e. All of the above

37) Regarding the biochemical properties of dopamine, all of the
 following statements are true, except:

 a. The rate-limiting step in the synthesis of any of the catecholamines is
 catalysed by tyrosine kinase
 b. Monoamine oxidase (MAO) is located on the outer mitochondrial
 membrane, principally in the presynaptic terminal
 c. Catechol-O-methyltransferase (COMT) is the principal enzyme
 metabolizing dopamine
 d. MAOB selectively metabolizes dopamine
 e. The primary metabolite of dopamine is homovanillic acid (HVA)

38) Peptide neurotransmitters include:

 a. Endogenous opioids
 b. Substance P
 c. Neurotensin
 d. Cholecystokinin
 e. All of the above

39) Regarding amino acid neurotransmitters, which of the following
 statements is true?

 a. GABA is an inhibitory amino acid
 b. Glutamate is an excitatory amino acid
 c. Benzodiazepines, barbiturates and several anticonvulsants act through
 GABAergic mechanisms
 d. Phencyclidine (PCP) acts at glutamate receptors
 e. All of the above

40) Which of the following is true of GABA?

 a. It does not cross the blood–brain barrier
 b. The highest concentrations are in the midbrain and the diencephalons
 c. It is synthesized from glutamate by the rate-limiting enzyme glutamic
 acid decarboxylase (GAD)
 d. Its synthesis requires pyridoxine as a cofactor
 e. All of the above

41) Which of the following statements is true regarding GABA receptors?

    a. The $GABA_B$ receptor is G-protein coupled

    b. $GABA_A$ and $GABA_C$ are directly acting, ligand-gated chloride ion channels that increase membrane polarization

    c. The $GABA_B$ agonist baclofen is used to treat spasticity

    d. The $GABA_A$ receptor antagonists bicuculline and picrotoxin induce seizures

    e. All of the above

42) All of the following anticonvulsants are correctly paired with their actions on GABA, except:

    a. Progabide–Hydrophobic GABA receptor agonist

    b. Tiagabine–Inhibits the GABA transporter

    c. Vigabatrin–Inhibits the GABA transporter

    d. Topiramate–Potentiates $GABA_A$ receptor activity

    e. Gabapentin–GABA receptor agonist

43) Glutamate is the primary neurotransmitter in all of the following areas of the brain, except:

    a. The cerebellar granule cells

    b. The striatum

    c. The intrinsic neurons for the inhibitory feedback loops

    d. The cells of the hippocampal molecular layer and entorhinal cortex

    e. The thalamospinal and corticospinal projections

44) Glutamate receptors include:

    a. The NMDA receptor

    b. The AMPA receptor

    c. The kinate receptor

    d. The AP4 receptor

    e. All of the above

45) All of the following statements are true regarding NMDA receptors, except:

    a. They allow the passage of sodium, potassium and calcium

    b. Their voltage-gated channels open only when bound by two molecules of glutamate and one molecule of glyceine

    c. NMDA receptor channels open when the membrane potential rises above 65 mV

    d. They are blocked by physiological concentrations of magnesium

    e. They are blocked by phencyclidine and dizocilpine

46) Regarding glutamate receptors, all of the following statements are true, except:

a. NMDA receptor antagonists have been shown to prevent the formation of memory
b. AMPA and kinate receptors share their principal effect with NMDA receptors
c. The AP4 receptor is an excitatory autoreceptor
d. The ACPD receptor is a metabotropic receptor
e. The ACPD receptor is G-protein coupled and exerts its effects through the phosphoinositol second messenger system

47) Regarding pathophysiology associated with glutamate, all of the following statements are correct, except:

a. Glutamate release is inhibited by nicotine
b. Excessive stimulation of glutamate receptors may cause excessive intraneuronal concentration of calcium and nitric oxide
c. Psychotomimetic effects of phencyclidine on glutamate receptors may explain the pathophysiology associated with schizophrenia
d. Dopamine and glutamate were observed to have opposing effects
e. Sensitivity of nigral dopamine-containing neurons to excitotoxicity may explain the involvement of glutamates in the pathophysiology associated with Parkinsonism

48) The blood-oxygen-level dependent (BOLD) sequence of the brain is obtained by:

a. Computerized tomography scans
b. Magnetic resonance spectroscopy
c. Functional magnetic resonance imaging
d. Single-photon emission computerized tomography
e. Positron emission tomography

49) ^{123}I-ioflupane-SPECT (single-photon emission computerized tomography) DaTSCAN is useful in the diagnosis of:

a. Frontotemporal dementia
b. Alzheimer's disease
c. Lewy body dementia
d. Vascular dementia
e. All of the above

50) Parkinson's disease occurs in a rare autosomal-dominant form caused by mutations in which of the following genes?

a. Alpha synuclein gene
b. UCHLI gene
c. NR4A2 gene
d. LRRK2 gene
e. All of the above

1) e.
Linkage studies have shown a relation between schizophrenia and the neuregulin-1 gene.

2) b.
Transcription is the transfer of information from DNA to tRNA.
Translation is the process of producing proteins from messenger RNA.

3) c.
The phenotype is transmitted only if both parents are homozygous in autosomal-recessive conditions, while in autosomal-dominant conditions it can be transmitted even if one parent is heterozygous.

4) b.
Males inherit their X chromosome from their mother, hence male-to-male transmission cannot occur. X-linked recessive disorders are rare.

5) c.
Molecular genetics are used to find the genes for specific diseases. For this, the DNA has to be cut or spliced at specific areas. Cutting, splicing, blotting and recombination are all techniques used in molecular genetics.

6) d.
Down syndrome relates to trisomy 21. Edwards syndrome relates to trisomy 18. Patau syndrome relates to trisomy 13.

7) c.
Marfan syndrome is an autosomal-dominant disorder. There are 46 autosomal chromosomes and any deformity in them usually is prevalent equally in both sexes.

8) c.
Concordance is seen in particular in studies of twins where both co-twins show the same disorder. A proband or index case is the affected person in a family risk study.

9) b.
Hurler syndrome is autosomal recessive.

10) c.
The prevalence of dementia increases with age. Around a third of the population over the age of 85 years suffer from dementia.

Ott A, Breteler MM, van Harskamp F, Claus JJ, van der Cammen TJ, Grobbee DE, Hofman A. Prevalence of Alzheimer's disease and vascular dementia: association with education. The Rotterdam study. *BMJ* 1995; 310: 970–3.

11) a.
Heritability is the difference in the concordance between monozygotic twins and dizygotic twins rather than the concordance in any one type of twins. Penetrance is the likelihood of a person with a genotype known to cause a phenotype presenting that characteristic.

12) e.
These are all findings from important studies on personality disorders except for choice **e**, which should have been that parents of antisocial children show more antisocial behaviour than do the biological parents of children who are not antisocial. References for answers **a** and **b** are Lyons *et al.* (1995), and **c**, Cadoret (1978). Refer to the personality disorder section in Gelder *et al.* (2006).

Cadoret RJ. Psychopathology in adopted-away offspring of biologic parents with antisocial behavior. *Arch Gen Psychiatry* 1978; 35: 176–84.
Gelder M, Harrison P, Cowen P. *Shorter Oxford Textbook of Psychiatry*, 5th edn. Oxford: Oxford University Press, 2006.
Lyons MJ, True WR, Eisen SA, *et al.* Differential heritability of adult and juvenile antisocial traits. *Arch Gen Psychiatry* 1995; 52: 906–15.

13) e.
A nucleoside is the nitrogenous base and sugar. A nucleotide is a nucleoside plus a phosphate. DNA and RNA are polymers.

14) a.
DNA strand synthesis always occur in the $5'-3'$ direction. Synthesis occurs in the other strand by production of Okazaki fragments. DNA ligase binds the Okazaki fragments together. Thymine is the nucleotide used instead of uracil in DNA. Uracil is the nucleotide used in RNA. Helicase helps in cutting of the hydrogen bonds holding the two DNA strands.

15) c.
Synthesis of DNA is semi-conservative, as on both identical daughter duplexes it has an original strand. Also, it is semi-discontinuous, as DNA is formed discontinuously on the lagging strand. Okazaki fragments are produced from the lagging strand and not from the leading strand.

16) e.
Family studies, twin studies and adoption studies are the conventional methods of genetic study, while modern methods include recombinant fraction, restriction endonucleases and linkage analysis.

17) d.
The most common type of Down syndrome (95%) arises because of meiotic non-dysjunction; less than 5% is due to translocation. Edwards syndrome is due to trisomy 18. Trisomy 13 leads to Patau syndrome. Prader–Willi syndrome is due to partial deletion of the long arm of chromosome 15. Deletion on chromosome 11 may lead to Wilms' tumour.

18) c.
Males with Klinefelter syndrome usually present with small testes and low testosterone level, and are hence infertile. They usually have gynaecomastia and elongated limbs. Often their IQ is normal.

19) a.
Turner syndrome is diagnosed by buccal mucosal cell chromosomal analysis showing XO. Girls with Turner syndrome usually have short stature. Cardiovascular defects include atrial septal defects and coarctation of the aorta.

20) b.
Fragile X syndrome is the most common cause of mental retardation in males after Down syndrome. All the others are features of fragile X syndrome.

21) e.
Caplan syndrome usually presents with rheumatoid disease plus pulmonary symptoms (pneumoconiosis). Tall stature and arachnodactyly are seen in Marfan syndrome.

22) c.
RNA splicing, capping and polyadenylation are all types of post-transcriptional processing. Transcription occurs in the $5'-3'$ direction. AUG is the initiation codon. Translation occurs after transcription.

23) b.
Duchenne muscular dystrophy is mainly seen in males since it is an X-linked disorder and females are usually carriers.

24) c.
Both artificial embryo twinning and somatic cell nuclear transfer are types of cloning used in laboratories. Artificial embryo twinning is very similar to the natural process of twin formation.

25) b.
One of the main differences between RNA and DNA is in the pyramidine bases. RNA has uracil in place of thymine as the pyramidine base in the nucleotides.

26) c.

The mutation occurs in the DHCR7 (7-dehydrocholesterol reductase) gene on chromosome 11. The autosomal-recessive disorder, which to date has no cure, can be supported only with cholesterol supplementation, owing to an increase in life expectancy. Those affected, however, are mentally retarded.

27) a.

Phenylketonuria is associated with low IQ.

28) b.

The incidence of classical galactosaemia is 55 000 to 60 000.

29) e.

The defective gene in cystic fibrosis is on chromosome 7.

30) a.

Alpha-1-antitrypsin deficiency is one of the most common genetic causes of liver disease in children.

31) e.

Heritability is the proportion of the liability to a disorder in a population that is accounted for by genetic effects; it is usually expressed as a percentage. It is highest for schizophrenia and bipolar disorder (80%); for alcohol problem or dependence it is 60%; for major depression and panic disorder it is 40% for each; and for generalized anxiety disorder it is 35%.

32) c.

Most polymorphisms have no known significance, especially those that are silent or conservative substitutions.

33) e.

In APOE4 in Alzheimer's disease and COMT Val158Met in schizophrenia the variants are coding, but in most genetic variations in psychiatric disorders they are non-coding. The non-coding variants may affect processing of mRNA.

34) e.

The limbic system (Papez circuit) was described by James Papez in 1937. In addition to **a** to **d**, the cingulate gyrus is also part of it.

35) d.

The peak of synaptogenesis occurs in the first two postnatal years; the thalamic axon first synapses to the subplate neurons, and in normal development the axon detaches from the subplate neurons and proceeds superficially to synapse on the true cortical cell. In normal development, the subplate neurons degenerate and the presence of heterotopic neurons within the frontal lobe and failure to complete axonal path finding are thought to be associated with pathology in schizophrenia.

36) e.
Substances that have been shown to meet only a few of the criteria are referred to as putative neurotransmitters.

37) c.
Monoamine oxidase (MAO) is the principal enzyme metabolizing dopamine; catechol-O-methyltransferase (COMT) metabolizes dopamine to a lesser extent.

38) e.
Peptide receptors are members of the seven-transmembrane domain, G-protein linked family. Almost all peptide neurotransmitters coexist in storage vesicles with other neurotransmitters.

39) e.
GABA and glutamate receptors are thought to be associated with anxiety disorders and schizophrenia.

40) e.
GABA is metabolized by enzyme GABA transaminase and is the primary neurotransmitter in the intrinsic neurons that function as local mediators for the inhibitory feedback loops.

41) e.
Because GABA is thought to suppress seizure activity, anxiety and mania, considerable effort has been devoted to synthesizing drugs that potentiate GABA activity.

42) e.
Gabapentin is a GABA derivative and an effective anticonvulsant, but it has no activity on GABA receptors or GABA transporters.

43) c.
Glutamate is an excitatory amino acid; glycine (an inhibitory amino acid) is the primary neurotransmitter in intrinsic neurons for the inhibitory feedback loops.

44) e.
There are five types of glutamate receptors: NMDA receptors; AMPA (alpha amino-3-hydroxy-5-methyl-4-isoxazolepropionic acid) receptors; kinate receptors; AP4 (1,2 amino-4-phosphorobutyrate) receptors; and CAPD (trans-1-aminocyclopentane-1-3-dicarboxylic acid) receptors.

45) c.
NMDA receptor channels open when the membrane potential rises above -65 mV.

46) c.
The AP4 receptor is an inhibitory autoreceptor.

47) a.
Nicotine stimulates the release of glutamate.

48) c.
Functional magnetic resonance imaging does not detect brain activity per se, but detects blood flow and levels of oxygenated haemoglobin in the blood as BOLD signals.

49) c.
DaTSCAN involves injection of an intravenous radiolabelled ligand of the presynaptic dopamine amine transporter (DaT) followed by SPECT using a gamma-camera; it evaluates the amount of presynaptic dopamine transporters in the striatum.

50) e.
There is also an autosomal-recessive form due to mutations in several other gene, including PARKIN, DJ1 and PNK1.

Further reading

Gelder M, Harrison P, Cowen P. *Shorter Oxford Textbook of Psychiatry*, 5th edn. Oxford: Oxford University Press, 2006.

Puri B, Hall A. *Revision Notes in Psychiatry*, 2nd edn. London: Arnold/ Hodder Education, 2004.

Sadock BJ, Sadock VA. *Kaplan and Sadock's Synopsis of Psychiatry*, 10th edn. Baltimore, MD: Lippincott Williams and Wilkins, 2008.

Stahl SM. *Stahl's Essential Psychopharmacology: Neuroscientific Basis and Practical Applications*, 3rd edn. Cambridge: Cambridge University Press, 2008.

6. Psychopharmacology: Questions

1) All of the following statements are true regarding cytochrome P450 enzymes, except:
   a. Most psychotherapeutic drugs are inactivated by CYP 450 enzymes by oxidation
   b. Persons with genetic polymorphisms in the CYP genes that encode inefficient versions of CYP enzymes are considered poor metabolizers
   c. The CYP enzymes act primarily in the endoplasmic reticulum of the hepatocytes and the cells of the intestine
   d. Viral hepatitis and cirrhosis affect the efficiency of drug metabolism by CYP enzymes
   e. About 25% of Caucasians have low levels of CYP enzymes and are poor metabolizers

2) Regarding hepatic enzymes, all of the following statements are true, except:
   a. Poor metabolizers are detected by their slow metabolism of debrisoquine or dextromethorphan
   b. Slow acetylators metabolize phenelzine slowly
   c. Slow acetylation is an autosomal-dominant trait
   d. Direct inhibition of hepatic enzymes is usually more profound than competitive inhibition
   e. Haloperidol inhibits the CYP 2D6 enzyme

3) Expression of CYP genes may be induced by all of the following, except:
   a. Alcohol
   b. Barbiturates
   c. Anticonvulsants
   d. Smoking
   e. Grapefruit juice

4) Cimetidine:
   a. Is an inhibitor of CYP 3A4
   b. Increases the metabolism of valproate
   c. May inhibit the metabolism and increase the plasma concentration of alprazolam
   d. Decreases the plasma concentration of mirtazapine and sertraline
   e. Increases the risk of ventricular arrhythmias when given with sertindole

5) Which of the following statements is true of polymorphic (allelic) variation in DNA?

a. It may produce proteins that interact with psychotropic drugs
b. It may modify the likelihood of therapeutic response
c. It may result in development of adverse reactions
d. It may affect blood levels of drugs and thereby brain exposure
e. All of the above

6) Pharmacogenetic studies in psychiatry have shown all of the following, except:

a. Mutations in the gene for CYP 2D6 may be associated with antipsychotic drug-induced tardive dyskinesia
b. Alleles associated with decreased expression of 5-HT transporters are associated with better response to SSRIs
c. Therapeutic response to clozapine may be associated with specific alleles of the 5-HT$_{2A}$ receptor
d. Weight gain with antipsychotic drugs is associated with an allele of the 5-HT$_{2C}$ receptor
e. The pathogenic mechanism of the most prominent genes in schizophrenia includes dysregulation of the NMDA glutamate receptor

7) According to current genetic research, the key genes that regulate neuronal connectivity and synaptogenesis in schizophrenia include:

a. BDNF
b. Dysbindin
c. Neuregulin
d. DISC-I
e. All of the above

8) Which of the following pharmacokinetic properties is not applicable to most psychotropic drugs?

a. Highly lipophilic
b. Largely protein bound
c. Small volume of distribution
d. Metabolized in the liver
e. Excreted mainly through the kidney

9) Which of the following statements is true about lithium?

a. It is filtered passively in the kidney and excretion is directly related to glomerular filtration rate (GFR)
b. Reabsorption occurs in the distal tubule in competition with sodium
c. Reabsorption increases when that of sodium is increased
d. Furosemide and thiazide diuretics decrease serum lithium levels
e. Lithium clearance is decreased in pregnancy

10) All of the following are known causes of significant elevation of lithium levels, except:

a. Thiazide diuretics
b. NSAIDs
c. Dehydration
d. Sodium restriction
e. Theophylline

11) Which of the following explains the mechanism of action of lithium?

a. Inositol depletion hypothesis
b. Inhibition of glycogen synthase kinase 3 (GSK-3)
c. Inhibition of protein kinase C
d. Modulation of G proteins
e. All of the above

12) All of the following statements are true regarding the prescription of psychotropic medications in pregnancy, except:

a. One meta-analysis has shown an increased risk of oral clefts after first-trimester exposure to benzodiazepines
b. If an antidepressant is required, it is probably better to use long-established preparations like imipramine and amitriptyline
c. There is a lower rate of congenital malformation in babies exposed to lower-potency antipsychotics such as chlorpromazine
d. Recent epidemiological studies have suggested that while the relative risk of Ebstein's anomaly is increased at least tenfold in infants exposed to lithium in the first trimester, the absolute risk is very low
e. The neural tube defect associated with anticonvulsants may be associated with folate metabolism

13) Neonatal complications are associated with treatment of psychiatric disorders with which of the following drugs in the later stages of pregnancy?

a. Tricyclic antidepressants
b. SSRIs
c. Lithium
d. Benzodiazepines
e. All of the above

14) All of the following are secreted in breast milk in significant amounts, except:

a. Benzodiazepines
b. Clozapine
c. Fluoxetine
d. Lithium
e. Valproate

15) Regarding the pharmacological properties of sedatives and hypnotics, all of the following statements are true, except:

    a. Absorption of lorazepam is poor following intramuscular injections and diazepam should be preferred in intramuscular use

    b. Benzodiazepine-sensitive $GABA_A$ receptor subtypes are thought to be post-synaptic in location

    c. Benzodiazepine and alcohol cross-tolerance is explained by similar action on the $GABA_A$ receptor

    d. Zolpidem and zaleplon selectively activate only one of the benzodiazepine-binding sites and they lack muscle-relaxant and anticonvulsant properties

    e. All the benzodiazepines produce a moderate decrease in REM sleep and are not associated with REM rebound

16) Which of the following statements is true of buspirone?

    a. It is effective in the treatment of panic disorder

    b. Anxiolytic effects develop within a few hours

    c. It is effective in treating benzodiazepine withdrawal

    d. It acts through benzodiazepine receptors

    e. It does not cause sedation

17) All of the following statements are true regarding benzodiazepine withdrawal, except:

    a. It generally begins within 7 days of stopping a long-acting benzodiazepine

    b. It is characterized by heightened sensitivity to perceptual stimuli and perceptual disturbances

    c. The symptoms generally last for 3–10 days

    d. It is more common with short-acting drugs than with ones with a longer half-life

    e. It can be effectively treated with flumazenil

18) Regarding the action of antipsychotic drugs on dopamine D2 receptors, all of the following statements are true, except:

    a. The blockade of D2 receptors in the mesolimbic pathway leads to a reduction in the positive symptoms of schizophrenia

    b. Impairment in the reward mechanism and the development of negative symptoms are associated more with blockade of D2 receptors in the mesocortical pathway than in the mesolimbic pathway

    c. The blockade of D2 receptors in the nigrostriatal pathway leads to extrapyramidal symptoms

    d. The blockade of D2 receptors in the tuberoinfundibular pathway is associated with galactorrhoea and amenorrhoea

    e. If D2 receptors in the nigrostriatal pathway are chronically blocked, this can produce tardive dyskinesia

19) Regarding serotonin dopamine antagonism, all of the following statements are correct, except:

a. 5-HT_{1A} receptors act as an accelerator for dopamine release
b. 5-HT_{2A} receptors act as a brake on dopamine release
c. 5-HT_{2C} receptors regulate dopamine and noradrenaline release and play a role in obesity, mood and cognition
d. 5-HT_3 receptors regulate excitatory interneurons
e. 5-HT_7 receptors may be involved in circadian rhythms

20) Which of the following statements is true regarding 5-HT_{2A} receptors?

a. They excite cortical pyramidal neurons
b. They increase glutamate release
c. They decrease dopamine release
d. They are involved in sleep and hallucinations
e. All of the above

21) Which of the following statements is true regarding 5-HT_{2A} antagonism?

a. It may reduce extrapyramidal symptoms (EPS)
b. It may reduce negative symptoms
c. It may improve positive symptoms
d. It may reduce hyperprolactinaemia
e. All of the above

22) Which drug is best described by the given pharmacological profile?

A potent antagonist at both 5-HT_2 receptors and dopamine D2 receptors. Also possesses alpha-1-adrenoceptor-blocking properties. Causes hyperprolactinaemia.

a. Risperidone
b. Olanzapine
c. Zotepine
d. Quetiapine
e. Aripiprazole

23) Which drug is best described by the given pharmacological profile?

Moderate D2-receptor-antagonist activity with anticholinergic and histamine H1 receptor-blocking property. Causes strong sedative effects, weight gain and abnormal glucose tolerance.

a. Risperidone
b. Olanzapine
c. Zotepine
d. Quetiapine
e. Aripiprazole

24) Which drug is best described by the given pharmacological profile?

5-H2D2 receptor antagonist also binding to $5\text{-}HT_{1A}$ receptors and acting as a noradrenaline reuptake inhibitor. Somnolence and dizziness are common side-effects and it causes relatively little weight gain.

a. Quetiapine
b. Aripiprazole
c. Ziprasidone
d. Zotepine
e. Bifeprunox

25) Which drug is best described by the given pharmacological profile?

Partial dopamine agonist that also has $5\text{-}HT_2$ receptor-blocking properties. It has side-effects like insomnia, nausea and vomiting. It is less likely to cause weight gain or significant extrapyramidal symptoms.

a. Sertindole
b. Paliperidone
c. Perospirone
d. Aripiprazole
e. Loxapine

26) All of the following statements regarding clozapine are true, except:

a. It is a potent D2 receptor antagonist
b. It blocks all types of dopamine receptors (D1–5)
c. According to positron emission tomography (PET) studies, it exerts its therapeutic effect while blocking 40–60% of D2 receptors in the striatum
d. It has agonist activity on the acetylcholine M4 receptor, leading to hypersalivation
e. It reduces the risk of suicide

27) Which of the following antipsychotic depot preparations has the longest duration of action?

a. Flupentixol decanoate
b. Haloperidol decanoate
c. Pipotiazine palmitate
d. Zuclopenthixol decanoate
e. Fluphenazine decanoate

28) All of the following statements regarding the pharmacological properties of psychotropic drugs are true, except:

   a. Amisulpride is excreted unchanged by the kidney and is regarded as safe in hepatic impairment
   b. Moclobemide is regarded as a safe choice of antidepressant in epilepsy
   c. Citalopram and sertraline are contraindicated in renal impairment
   d. Pimozide and thioridazine increase the QT interval
   e. Clozapine should not be given with carbamazepine, co-trimoxazole or penicillamine, as it may cause agranulocytosis

29) All of the following are important mechanisms of action of antidepressants, except:

   a. Stimulation of inhibitory autoreceptors in the midbrain
   b. Autoreceptors of NA and 5-HT neurons become subsensitive
   c. Increased monoamine function leading to activation of second messengers
   d. Synaptic plasticity and remodelling
   e. All of the above

30) Which of the following antidepressants causes significant blockade of dopamine D2 receptors?

   a. Amoxapine
   b. Clomipramine
   c. Lofepramine
   d. Maprotiline
   e. Mianserin

31) All of the following side-effects are paired correctly with the antidepressant drug known to cause them, except:

   a. Mianserin–Cognitive impairment
   b. Lofepramine–Hepatitis
   c. Maprotiline–Higher incidence of seizures
   d. Amitriptyline–Insomnia
   e. Dothiepin–Sedation

32) Which of the following statements is true of tricyclic antidepressants?

   a. They antagonize the hypertensive effects of alpha-2 adrenoceptor agonists such as clonidine
   b. They are not safe to combine with thiazides and ACE inhibitors
   c. They are safe to use with amiodarone
   d. They may decrease the action of warfarin
   e. Plasma level can be decreased by cimetidine

33) Regarding the pharmacological properties of SSRIs, all of the following statements are true, except:

   a. Gastrointestinal side-effects are common
   b. Paroxetine is associated with acute dystonia in the first few days of treatment
   c. Ejaculatory delay and anorgasmia are common side-effects
   d. They are more cardiotoxic than tricyclic antidepressants
   e. Serotonin toxicity can occur when they are combined with MAOIs or sumatriptan

34) Fluoxetine causes significant inhibition of all CYP enzymes, except:

   a. CYP 1A2
   b. CYP 2D6
   c. CYP 2C9
   d. CYP 2C19
   e. CYP 3A/4

35) Which of the following is a reversible MAO-A inhibitor?

   a. Phenelzine
   b. Tranylcypromine
   c. Amphetamine
   d. Isocarboxazid
   e. Moclobemide

36) Regarding the pharmacological properties of antidepressants, all of the following statements are true, except:

   a. Reboxetine is a substrate of CYP 3A
   b. Reboxetine causes urinary incontinence
   c. Venlafaxine produces potent blockade of 5-HT reuptake with lesser effects on noradrenaline
   d. Venlafaxine causes somnolence
   e. Duloxetine is five times more potent in inhibiting the reuptake of 5-HT than that of noradrenaline

37) Regarding mood stabilizers, all of the following statements are true, except:

   a. Valproate may be more effective than lithium in mixed affective states
   b. Lamotrigine blocks sodium channels and reduces the release of glutamate
   c. One of the most common side-effects of gabapentin is insomnia
   d. A combination of lamotrigine and gabapentin can cause neurotoxicity
   e. Gabapentin is not metabolized in the kidney and is excreted entirely by the kidney

38) All of the following statements regarding psychostimulants are true, except:

   a. In adults, the agreed indication for amphetamine is narcolepsy
   b. Methylphenidate is approved for use in attention deficit hyperactivity disorder (ADHD) in children
   c. Modafinil increases the release and blocks the reuptake of dopamine and noradrenaline
   d. Modafinil is licensed for the treatment of narcolepsy
   e. Amphetamines can cause severe hypertension when used with MAOIs

39) Regarding pharmacological treatments to help maintenance of abstinence from alcohol, all of the following statements are true, except:

   a. Disulfiram acts by blocking oxidation of alcohol and accumulating acetaldehyde, causing an unpleasant reaction
   b. Disulfiram is safe to use in patients with cardiac problems
   c. Acamprosate is believed to act by stimulating GABA inhibitory neurotransmission and decreasing the effects of glutamate
   d. Adverse effects of acamprosate include diarrhoea
   e. Naltrexone is believed to block the reinforcing effects of alcohol

40) Which of the following drugs is useful in planned withdrawal of opioids?

   a. Loperamide
   b. Metoclopramide
   c. Non-steroidal analgesics
   d. Lofexidine
   e. All of the above

41) All of the following statements regarding the pharmacological management of opioid withdrawal are true, except:

   a. In short-term non-opioid treatment, an alpha-2 agonist is recommended
   b. In short-term treatment, buprenorphine is found to produce a better outcome than clonidine
   c. It is recommended to start methadone in a higher dose and lower it gradually, titrating against the presence of withdrawal symptoms
   d. Methadone may be preferable in pregnancy because of greater experience with its use
   e. Naltrexone treatment has a role in certain dependent subjects with high motivation

42) Bupropion is found to be useful in which of the following?

a. Depression
b. Attention deficit hyperactivity disorder (ADHD)
c. Cocaine detoxification
d. Smoking cessation
e. All of the above

43) All of the following statements regarding sibutramine are true, except:

a. It is a potent antidepressant
b. It is used as an appetite suppressant to treat obesity
c. It is a reuptake inhibitor of serotonin
d. It may cause dry mouth and constipation
e. It may exacerbate narrow-angle glaucoma

44) All of the following statements regarding sildenafil are true, except:

a. It is a non-selective phosphodiesterase inhibitor
b. It is effective in erectile dysfunction
c. It may reverse SSRI-induced anorgasmia in both men and women
d. It is contraindicated in pulmonary artery hypertension
e. It is contraindicated in people taking organic nitrates in any form

45) Which of the following statements is true of yohimbine?

a. It is an alpha-2 adrenergic receptor antagonist
b. It is used to treat both idiopathic and medication-induced male sexual dysfunction
c. It may cause hypertension
d. It blocks the effects of clonidine
e. All of the above

46) Regarding the use of antipsychotic drug treatment and behavioural and psychotic symptoms in dementia, all of the following statements are true, except:

a. Haloperidol may be useful in reducing aggression
b. Risperidone and olanzapine were not found to be useful in reducing aggression
c. The evidence suggests that the increased risk of stroke is shared by all antipsychotics
d. Antipsychotics can precipitate an irreversible and fatal syndrome of Parkinsonism in people with Lewy body dementia
e. Antipsychotics may hasten cognitive decline

47) Regarding the pharmacological properties of drugs used in the treatment of dementia, all of the following statements are true, except:

a. Tacrine is a cholinesterase inhibitor with a favourable side-effect profile for use with elderly people
b. Donepezil is a reversible long-acting selective inhibitor of acetylcholinesterase without inhibition of butyrylcholinesterase
c. In addition to causing an irreversible inhibition of acetylcholinesterase, rivastigmine inhibits butyrylcholinesterase
d. Galantamine inhibits acetylcholinesterase with positive allosteric modification of nicotinic cholinergic receptors
e. Memantine is an uncompetitive open-channel NMDA receptor antagonist with low to moderate affinity

48) Which of the following is a disease-modifying agent in development that acts on amyloid processing in Alzheimer's disease?

a. Immunotherapy using ACC 001
b. Beta amyloid antagonists (tramiprosate)
c. Gamma secretase inhibitors SCH1390499
d. Gamma secretase modulator (flurizan)
e. All of the above

49) All of the following statements regarding dopamine receptors in the brain are true, except:

a. D1 and D5 stimulate adenylate cyclase to form cyclic AMP as a second messenger
b. D2, D3 and D4 are more common in the limbic areas than in the caudate–putamen region
c. The five subtypes of dopamine receptors have common amino acid sequences and are associated with the same chromosome
d. Antipsychotic drugs, by blocking dopamine receptors, lead initially to an increased firing rate of nigrostriatal and mesolimbic but not mesocortical dopaminergic neurons
e. Different variants of the D2 receptor exist

50) Regarding 5-HT receptors, all of the following statements are true, except:

a. All classes of 5-HT receptors are metabotropic receptors
b. 5-HT_1 receptors are mainly cell body autoreceptors
c. Buspirone is an agonist and pindolol is an antagonist on 5-HT_{1A} receptors
d. Sumatriptan is an agonist of both 5-HT_{1B} and 5-HT_{1D}
e. 5-HT_{2A} receptors facilitate excitatory effects on cortical and other neurons

6. Psychopharmacology: Answers

1) e.
About 7–10% of Caucasians have low levels of CYP enzymes and are poor metabolizers.

2) c.
Slow acetylation is an autosomal-recessive trait. CYP 2D6, IA2, 2C, 3A3/4 are important CYP enzymes that metabolize psychotropic drugs.

3) e.
Grapefruit juice appears to inhibit CYP 3A4 activity in the gut mucosa.

4) e.
Cimetidine is an inducer of CYP 3A4; it inhibits the metabolism of valproate, carbamazepine and phenytoin; it may increase the metabolism and decrease the plasma concentration of alprazolam, which is a substrate of CYP 3A4; it increases the plasma concentration of mirtazapine, sertraline, meclobamide and tricyclics.

5) e.
Polymorphic (allelic) variation in DNA may result in the production of proteins that interact with psychotropic drugs in different ways. Genetic variation in CYP-metabolizing enzymes can affect blood levels of drugs and thereby brain exposure.

6) b.
Alleles associated with decreased expression of 5-HT transporters are associated with poorer response to SSRIs.

7) e.
BDNF is brain-derived neurotrophic factor, which is a known trophic factor. Dysbindin, also known as dystrobrevin-binding protein 1, is involved in the formation of synaptic structures; neuregulin is involved in neuronal migration and in the genesis of glial cells and subsequent myelination of neurons by these cells; DISC-1 (disrupted in schizophrenia 1) is a disrupted gene linked to schizophrenia that makes a protein involved in neurogenesis, neuronal migration and dendritic organization.

8) c.
Because most of the psychotropic drugs are lipophilic, they tend to enter fat stores, from where they are released slowly, and they tend to have a large volume of distribution.

9) a.

Reabsorption of lithium occurs in the proximal tubule in competition with sodium. Lithium is also reabsorbed in the loop of Henle to a lesser extent but unlike sodium it is not further reabsorbed in the distal tubule, thus its excretion is not facilitated by diuretics such as thiazides acting at the distal tubule. Because proximal absorption is competitive with sodium, reabsorption of lithium increases when that of sodium is decreased. Conditions that increase glomerular filtration rate (GFR), such as pregnancy, increase lithium clearance.

10) e.

Frusemide is the safest diuretic as it acts in the loop of Henle and adequately blocks lithium reabsorption, generally without increasing the level. However, in all diuretic therapy, monitoring is required as it may cause sodium depletion. Aspirin and sulindac are the safest NSAIDs in lithium therapy. Theophylline decreases lithium levels.

11) e.

The pharmacological action of lithium is thought to be through a second messenger system such as the phosphatidylinositol system, where lithium inhibits the enzyme inositol monophosphate, modulates G proteins and, according to recent studies, regulates gene expression of growth factors and neuronal plasticity by interaction with downstream signal transduction cascades including GSK-3 and protein kinase C.

12) c.

Fluoxetine is not associated with increased risk of malformations. High-potency antipsychotics such as haloperidol are not associated with an increased risk of foetal abnormalities; however, there is a higher rate of congenital malformations in babies exposed to lower-potency antipsychotics such as chlorpromazine. Absolute risk of Ebstein's anomaly in infants exposed to lithium is between 0.05 and 0.1. The neural tube defect associated with anticonvulsants may be associated with folate metabolism but the role of folate treatment in their prevention has not been established.

13) e.

Tricyclic antidepressants are associated with withdrawal reactions in neonates. SSRIs may be associated with complications such as jitteriness, hypoglycaemia and respiratory difficulties. Lithium causes floppy baby syndrome.

14) e.

The amounts of valproate and carbamazepine are considered to be too low to be harmful.

15) a.

Absorption of lorazepam and midazolam are rapid following intramuscular injections and that of diazepam is poor; the former should be preferred in intramuscular use.

16) e.

Buspirone is an azapirone effective in the treatment of generalized anxiety disorder but is not helpful in the treatment of panic disorder. The anxiolytic effects take several days to develop and it cannot be used to treat benzodiazepine withdrawal. It acts on 5-HT_{1A} receptors.

17) e.

Flumazenil is a benzodiazepine antagonist, useful in reversing acute toxicity produced by benzodiazepines, but carries a risk of provoking acute benzodiazepine withdrawal.

18) b.

The density of D2 receptors is much lower in the cortex; the impairment in the reward mechanism and the development of negative symptoms are more associated with blockade of D2 receptors in the mesolimbic rather than the mesocortical pathway. Blockade of D2 receptors in the mesocortical pathway is also related to cognitive symptoms, negative symptoms and affective symptoms of schizophrenia.

19) d.

5-HT_3 receptors regulate inhibitory interneurons in the brain and also mediate vomiting via the vagal nerve. 5-HT_6 receptors may regulate release of neurotrophic factors.

20) e.

5-HT_{2A} receptors act as a dopamine (DA) brake. When 5-HT binds to 5-HT_{2A} receptors on post-synaptic DA neurons, this inhibits DA release. When 5-HT binds to 5-HT_{2A} receptors on GABA interneurons, this causes GABA release, which in turn inhibits DA release.

21) e.

The 5-HT_{2A} 'dopamine brake' action is disrupted by an antagonist (atypical antipsychotic) stimulating dopamine release in different pathways, resulting in these actions.

22) a.

Risperidone is a benzisoxazole. It has less affinity to D3 and D4 receptors, and blocks H1, alpha-1 and alpha-2 adrenoceptors but not actylcholine receptors. It may cause extrapyramidal symptoms (EPS), postural hypotension and sexual dysfunction.

23) b.
Olanzapine is a thienobenzodiazepine; adverse effects include oedema, hypotension, dry mouth and constipation.

24) c.
Ziprasidone has a tendency to increase the QT interval and is currently not licensed in the UK.

25) d.
Aripiprazole is less likely to cause extrapyramidal symptoms (EPS) and increased prolactin levels; other side-effects include agitation and insomnia.

26) a.
Clozapine is a weak dopamine D2 receptor antagonist but has a high affinity for 5-HT$_2$ receptors.

27) c.
Time to peak plasma level of pipotiazine palmitate is 9–10 days and frequency of administration is every four weeks. Zuclopenthixol has a shorter duration of action.

28) c.
Citalopram and sertraline are regarded as reasonable choices in renal impairment.

29) e.
Elaboration of neurotrophic factors is also thought to be a mechanism of action.

30) a.
Amoxapine is also an inhibitor of noradrenaline uptake. It may cause EPS and hyperprolactinaemia.

31) d.
Amitriptyline causes sedation and drowsiness.

32) a.
It is usually safe to combine tricyclic antidepressants with thiazides and ACE inhibitors; they are not safe to use with amiodarone; they may increase the action of warfarin; cimetidine increases the plasma levels of tricyclics.

33) d.
SSRIs are less cardiotoxic than tricyclics and they lack anticholinergic effects.

34) a.

CYP 1A2 inhibitors are fluoxamine and duloxetine; substrates include olanzapine, clozapine, haloperidol, tricyclic antidepressants and theophylline.

35) e.

Moclobemide does not have significant interactions with foodstuffs. It is reversible with a shorter half-life.

36) b.

Common side-effects of reboxetine are characteristic of cholinergic receptor blockade, through interaction of noradrenergic and cholinergic pathways. The most common ones include dry mouth, constipation, sweating, insomnia, urinary hesitancy, impotence and tachycardia.

37) c.

The most common side-effects of gabapentin include somnolence, dizziness, fatigue and nystagmus.

38) c.

Most of the psychostimulants increase the release and block the reuptake of dopamine and noradrenaline, but modafinil increases alertness and decreases sleepiness, apparently through non-catecholaminergic mechanisms. The precise mechanism of action of modafinil is unknown, although it is found to cause release of histamine and orexin in the tuberomammillary nucleus and lateral hypothalamus. It also has actions on dopamine transporters.

39) b.

The main contraindications for disulfiram are a history of heart failure, coronary artery disease, hypertension, psychosis and pregnancy.

40) e.

Loperamide and metoclopramide can be useful for gastrointestinal symptoms. NSAIDs can be useful for aches and pains. The alpha-2 adrenoceptor agonist lofexidine is as effective as methadone in ameliorating the withdrawal syndrome.

41) c.

There is a potential for methadone toxicity in patients whose tolerance is unknown or hard to assess. It is better to start with lower doses (not more than 40 mg daily) and increase them over a number of weeks, titrating against the presence of withdrawal symptoms.

42) e.

Bupropion is a unicyclic aminoketone-resembling amphetamine. Its common uses are in depression and smoking cessation and as a second-line treatment in attention deficit hyperactivity disorder (ADHD). Some clinicians recommend its use in cocaine detoxification.

43) a.
Sibutramine is a reuptake inhibitor of serotonin, noradrenaline and, to a lesser extent, dopamine, but it lacks any clinical antidepressant effect.

44) d.
Sildenafil is licensed for the treatment of some kinds of pulmonary hypertension. The most important potential adverse effect associated with sildenafil is myocardial infarction.

45) e.
Sildenafil and alprostadil are generally considered more efficacious for the treatment of male sexual dysfunction.

46) b.
One review of randomized controlled trials suggested that risperidone and olanzapine were effective in reducing aggression.

Sink KM, Holden KF, Yaffe K. Pharmacological treatment of neuropsychiatric symptoms of dementia: a review of the evidence. *JAMA* 2005; **293**: 596–608.

47) c.
Rivastigmine is a pseudoirreversible (it reverses itself over hours) inhibitor of acetylcholinesterase; rivastigmine inhibits butyrylcholinesterase within the glia.

48) e.
Positive tests of amyloid vaccines in animals have led to early clinical trials. These found evidence not only of stabilization of memory in Alzheimer's patients but also, perhaps more importantly, that amyloid plaques were removed.

49) c.
The five subtypes of dopamine receptors have different amino acid sequences and are associated with four different chromosomes.

50) a.
All classes of 5-HT receptors except 5-HT_3 are metabotropic (G-protein-linked) receptors.

Further reading

British National Formulary. *BNF 57*. London: Pharmaceutical Press. Also available at: www.bnf.org/bnf.

Cookson J, Taylor D, Katona C. *Use of Drugs in Psychiatry*, 5th edn. London: Gaskell, 2002.

Gelder M, Andreasen N, Lopez-Ibor J, Geddes J. Chapter 21. In: *New Oxford Textbook of Psychiatry*, 2nd edn. Oxford: Oxford University Press, 2009.

Rosenbaum JF, Arana GW, Hyman SE, *et al*. *Handbook of Psychiatric Drug Therapy*, 5th edn. Baltimore, MD: Lippincott Williams and Wilkins, 2005.

Sadock BJ, Sadock VA. Chapter 36. In: *Kaplan and Sadock's Synopsis of Psychiatry*, 10th edn. Baltimore, MD: Lippincott Williams and Wilkins, 2008.

Stahl SM. *Stahl's Essential Psychopharmacology: Neuroscientific Basis and Practical Applications*, 3rd edn. Cambridge: Cambridge University Press, 2008.

7. Epidemiology: Questions

1) Which of the following research methods is considered to have the highest credibility?

    a. Case reports
    b. Prospective studies
    c. Cross-sectional studies
    d. Retrospective studies
    e. Case series

2) Which of the following is likely to be the best guide for evidence-based practice?

    a. Randomized double-blind placebo-controlled trials
    b. Cross-sectional studies
    c. Retrospective studies
    d. Meta-analysis of randomized double-blind placebo-controlled trials
    e. Review articles

3) In epidemiological studies, which of the following is not used as a method to compensate for confounding variables?

    a. Recruitment
    b. Standardization
    c. Randomization
    d. Matching
    e. Modelling

4) Which of the following statements best explains the meaning of 'number needed to treat'?

    a. It explains the benefit for treating a large number of people
    b. It means that treating a minimum number of people can be of some benefit
    c. It expresses the benefit of an active treatment over placebo
    d. It expresses the benefit of placebo over an active treatment
    e. None of the above

5) Which of the following statements best describes the 'positive predictive value' of a screening instrument?

    a. The proportion of positive results that are truly positive
    b. The sum of all the positive results
    c. The proportion of negative results that are truly negative
    d. The sum of all negative results
    e. None of the above

6) The lifetime risk for a major depressive disorder in women in the Western world is:

  a. One in two
  b. One in four
  c. One in six
  d. One in eight
  e. One in ten

7) What is the annual incidence of schizophrenia?

  a. 1–2 per 100 000 population
  b. 5–10 per 100 000 population
  c. 10–20 per 100 000 population
  d. 100 per 100 000 population
  e. 200 per 100 000 population

8) Which of the following statements is true regarding suicide?

  a. Suicide rates are highest in young women
  b. Suicide rates are highest in young men
  c. Suicide rates are highest in older women
  d. Suicide rates are highest in older men
  e. There is no age or gender difference in suicide rates

9) Epidemiologically, which of the following groups of people has a higher rate of schizophrenia than the general population?

  a. Children with a biological parent suffering from schizophrenia
  b. Children with a first-degree relative suffering from schizophrenia
  c. Adopted children with a foster parent suffering from schizophrenia
  d. Adopted children with a biological parent suffering from schizophrenia
  e. Adopted children with a foster sibling suffering from schizophrenia

10) Incidence can be defined as:

  a. The number of new cases of illness at a given point in time
  b. The number of new cases occurring in a population over a designated period of time
  c. The number of hospital admissions during a designated time period
  d. The number of deaths during a designated time period
  e. The number of beds occupied in a hospital over a designated period of time

11) Prevalence can be defined as:

a. The total number of new cases reported in a designated period of time
b. The total number of treated cases in a population in a designated period of time
c. All new and pre-existing cases during a given period of time in a population
d. The total number of resistant cases of an illness in a population
e. The total number of hospital admissions due to a particular disease in a given population

12) Which of the following statements is not true about point prevalence?

a. It is a snapshot look at the population with regard to a particular disease
b. It is the number of people with a particular disease on a particular date
c. It includes both new and pre-existing cases
d. It is not similar to incidence
e. It is the number of people with a particular illness at any time during a specific time interval

13) In a population of 5000 people surveyed for psychosis, a prevalence rate of 7 per 1000 in 12 months was reported. What does it mean?

a. Seven new cases per 1000 population every year
b. Seven referrals to psychiatric services per 1000 population every year
c. A total of seven cases of psychosis per 1000 population every year
d. Seven treated cases of psychosis per 1000 population every year
e. Seven old cases of psychosis per 1000 population every year

14) Suppose an epidemiological study of relapse of psychotic illness and cannabis use reports a relative risk of 4.41 in cannabis users. What does it mean?

a. The relapsed cases are 4.41 times more likely to have had exposure to cannabis
b. Those with exposure to cannabis are 4.41 times more likely to have a relapse
c. People smoking cannabis are 4.41 times more likely to develop psychosis
d. Banning the use of cannabis is likely to reduce the incidence of psychosis by 4.41 times
e. There is no increased risk of a relapse of psychosis in people using cannabis

15) Suppose an epidemiological study looking at severe head injury and cognitive decline reports an odd ratio of 5.44 in the exposed population. What does this mean?

   a. People with cognitive decline are 5.44 times more likely to have had a severe head injury compared with those without cognitive decline
   b. People involved in severe head injuries are 5.44 times more likely to develop cognitive decline
   c. Cognitive decline after a severe head injury is inevitable
   d. Severe head injuries are the most common cause of cognitive decline
   e. People who have suffered from a head injury more than five times will always develop cognitive decline

16) Which one of the following statements is not true regarding the reliability of an instrument?

   a. It is concerned with the accuracy of its measurement
   b. It is high if the rating of the same instrument by other raters is similar
   c. It is high if its measurements accord with those of other instruments supposed to have the same function
   d. It concerns the reliability of its measurements
   e. It is high if the results are similar when the instrument is administered at two different time points

17) Which of the following measures is best suited to picking out the leading causes of death in a specific population?

   a. Mortality rates
   b. Crude death rate
   c. Incidence
   d. Proportional mortality
   e. Prevalence

18) The following formula can be used to calculate both incidence and prevalence for a specified time period:

$$\frac{X}{Y} \times 10n$$

Which of the following determines the primary difference between incidence and prevalence?

   a. X
   b. Y
   c. 10n
   d. The time period
   e. None of the above

19) An epidemiological study was conducted on two different types of cancers (A and B). It was found that the prevalence of cancer A was higher than that of cancer B but the incidence of both diseases was similar. Which of the following explanations could be responsible for these findings?

a. Patients recover more quickly from cancer A than from cancer B
b. Patients recover more quickly from cancer B than from cancer A
c. Patients die more quickly from cancer A than from cancer B
d. Patients with cancer A are not being treated properly
e. None of the above

20) To investigate the association between dementia and stroke, investigators conducted a case-control study of 100 cases (people with dementia) and 100 controls (people without dementia). Among the dementia cases, 50 had a history of stroke. Among those without dementia, 25 had a history of stroke. For this study, the odds ratio is:

a. 1.0
b. 1.5
c. 2.0
d. 3.0
e. It cannot be calculated from the given information

21) Which measure, relating to the epidemiology of schizophrenia, is the following equation likely to calculate?

$$\frac{\text{Number of patients in UK on 1 January 2010}}{\text{Total population of UK on 1 January 2010}} = ?$$

a. Incidence rate
b. Attack rate
c. Person time rate
d. Period prevalence
e. Point prevalence

22) All of the following statements are true regarding the use of psychiatric screening instruments in a general hospital setting, except:

a. They are used to detect uncommon syndromes
b. They should have cut-off scores based on sensitivity
c. They require normal distribution of scores
d. They include the CAGE questionnaire
e. They include the Geriatric Depression Scale

23) Which of the following statements is not true regarding rating scales in psychiatry?

a. Rating scales convert descriptive information into numerical data
b. The scores of rating scales cannot be used for inclusion or exclusion from a study
c. Rating scales can have cultural bias
d. The Brief Psychiatric Rating Scale (BPRS) measures positive symptoms
e. There are separate Hamilton rating scales for anxiety and depression

24) Which of the following is not a commonly used epidemiological study design?

a. Case-control study
b. Cross-sectional cohort survey
c. Ecological study
d. Randomized controlled trial
e. Systematic review

25) Which of the following is not a possible source of bias in epidemiological studies?

a. The procedure of matching controls to individual cases
b. Use of a measurement of exposure not independent of presence of disease
c. Retrospective exposure assessment
d. Adequate selection of controls
e. Effort after meaning

26) All of the following statements are true regarding confounding variables in epidemiological research, except:

a. They can be either a risk factor or a protective factor
b. They can be associated with both exposure and disease
c. They can be taken into account by introducing randomization in a study design
d. They are on the causal pathway between exposure and disease
e. They can be taken into account by introducing matching into a study design

27) Which of the following statements is not true regarding case-control studies?

a. They are experimental studies
b. They compare a group of cases with a group of controls
c. They can indicate possible risk factors for an illness
d. Odds ratios can be estimated from these studies
e. They cannot by themselves prove causality

28) Which of the following is not a rating scale for depression?

    a. HRSD
    b. BPRS
    c. MADRS
    d. BDI
    e. HADS

29) Which of the following statements is not true regarding confounding variables in epidemiological studies?

    a. They can lead to a spurious association
    b. They can be an independent risk factor for the disease
    c. They can never be a protective factor for the disease
    d. They can be adjusted by randomization
    e. They can be adjusted by matching

30) Which of the following statements is not true regarding reliability?

    a. It implies diagnostic consistency
    b. High reliability implies high validity
    c. It relates to the agreement between tests done on different occasions
    d. It relates to the agreement between raters
    e. It can be estimated by assessing test–retest reliability

31) Which of the following statements is not true regarding validity?

    a. The validity of diagnosis cannot be assessed by comparison with a gold standard
    b. Criterion validity means how valid the diagnosis is when judged against one or more external validators
    c. Face validity looks at whether the criteria used overtly relate to the diagnosis
    d. Construct validity looks at the conceptual soundness of the diagnosis and its consistency with available data
    e. Predictive validity looks at whether the diagnosis can be used to accurately predict outcome or other patient-related events

32) Which of the following statements is not true regarding the sensitivity and specificity of an instrument?

    a. The sensitivity of an instrument is the probability of diagnosing a disease when present
    b. The specificity of an instrument is the probability of not diagnosing a disease when present
    c. It is not possible for an instrument to be highly sensitive and highly specific
    d. Sensitivity increases as the threshold for making the diagnosis is lowered
    e. The specificity reduces as the threshold for making the diagnosis is lowered

33) Regarding the epidemiology of schizophrenia, all of the following statements are true, except:

a. Incidence is between 15 and 30 new cases per 100 000
b. Point prevalence is approximately 1%
c. Lifetime risk is approximately 1%
d. Age of onset is earlier in men than women
e. It is more common in males than females

34) Regarding the epidemiology of schizophrenia, which of the following statements is true?

a. Rates from urban areas are usually lower than those from rural areas
b. According to social drift theory, women are more likely to drift into inner-city areas
c. Social residue theory explains that healthy people migrate away from undesirable areas, leaving schizophrenics behind
d. Breeder hypothesis rejects environmental factors of aetiological importance in schizophrenia
e. There is a higher incidence in those who have married

35) Regarding the epidemiology of delusional disorders, all of the following statements are correct according to Munro's (1991) observations, except:

a. The mean age of onset is lower in males
b. The sex ratio is equal
c. The probability of delusional disorders is increased if there is a family history of delusional disorder and schizophrenia
d. Introverted personalities with long-standing interpersonal difficulties are more likely to suffer from delusional disorders
e. Delusional disorders increase with high rates of marital breakdown

36) Which of the following statements is true regarding depressive disorder?

a. It is more common in females in all age groups
b. The point prevalence is higher in men
c. The average age of onset is around the late thirties
d. The incidence is lower in those who are unmarried
e. There is a higher prevalence in middle-class than in working-class women

37) Which of the following statements is true regarding bipolar mood disorder?

a. The sex ratio is equal
b. The average age of onset is around the mid-twenties
c. It is more common in the upper social class
d. The point prevalence is between 0.4% and 1.25% in the adult population
e. All of the above

38) Suicide is more common in:

a. Men
b. People aged over 45
c. Divorced people
d. Social classes 1 and 4
e. All of the above

39) Deliberate self-harm is more common in:

a. Females
b. Those aged below 35
c. Divorced and single people
d. Lower social class
e. All of the above

40) In agoraphobias, there is a higher rate of comorbidity with:

a. Depression
b. Alcohol abuse
c. Simple phobia
d. Social phobia
e. All of the above

41) All of the following statements are true regarding the epidemiology of panic disorder, except:

a. It is twice as common in females as in males
b. Only the higher socioeconomic groups are affected
c. Onset is rare after the age of 40
d. It is more common in divorced people
e. A family history of panic disorder is associated with increased risk

42) All of the following statements are true regarding the epidemiology of generalized anxiety disorder (GAD), except:

a. Age of onset is earlier than in other anxiety disorders
b. Early-onset GAD is more likely in males
c. Early-onset GAD is associated with childhood fears
d. Early-onset GAD is associated with marital and sexual dysfunction
e. Late-onset GAD is more associated with stressful life events

43) Regarding the epidemiology of obsessive compulsive disorder, which of the following statements is true?

a. It is very rare in children
b. The sex ratio is equal
c. There is a bimodal age of onset
d. There is a decline in onset after the age of 35
e. All of the above

44) Regarding cyclical premenstrual symptoms, which of the following statements is true?

a. There is a higher prevalence in those around the age of 30 years
b. Prevalence decreases with increasing parity
c. There is a higher prevalence in women whose cycles are modified with oral contraceptive pills
d. There is a higher prevalence in women whose cycles are interrupted with pregnancy
e. All of the above

45) All of the following factors are associated with women who develop puerperal psychosis, except:

a. Increased rate of caesarean section
b. Lower social class
c. Older age at birth of first child
d. Primiparae
e. Previous history of manic depressive illness

46) All of the following statements regarding anorexia nervosa are true, except:

a. It is rare, with a prevalence of one to two per 1000 women
b. Peak age is 15–19 years
c. There is a higher prevalence in higher socioeconomic classes
d. There is a significant association with lower parental education
e. Incidence is 10 times higher in females than in males

47) Which of the following statements is true regarding bulimia?

a. Its prevalence may be slightly higher than that of anorexia
b. Social class distribution is more even than in anorexia
c. The age of onset is slightly higher than that of anorexia
d. The female to male ratio is 10:1
e. All of the above

48) Which of the following psychiatric morbidities has the highest prevalence among those aged over 65?

a. Dementia
b. Depression
c. Phobic disorders
d. Paranoid states
e. Personality disorders

49) Which of the following statements is true of Huntington's disease?

a. It is autosomal dominant and fully penetrant
b. It affects 50% of offspring
c. There are five cases per 100 000 in the UK
d. Onset is usually between the ages of 35 and 45 years
e. All of the above

50) Which of the following statements is true regarding late-onset psychosis?

a. It is more common in females
b. 46% have at least one Schneiderian first-rank symptom
c. The annual incidence is 17–26 per 100 000
d. It is associated with a lower rate of marriage and low fecundity
e. All of the above

7. Epidemiology: Answers

1) b.

Prospective studies are considered to have the highest credibility when compared to the other types of studies mentioned. The gold standards, however, are the randomized placebo-controlled trials.

2) d.

Meta-analysis of a number of randomized double-blind placebo-controlled trials is considered to be the best possible guide for evidence-based practice. They are considered more effective than individual randomized double-blind placebo-controlled trials.

3) a.

All the other four methods are commonly used to compensate for confounding variables such as age and sex.

4) c.

The 'number needed to treat' expresses the benefit of an active treatment over placebo. It is not only useful in explaining the outcome of a trial but it can also be used while making individual treatment decisions.

5) a.

The positive predictive value is the proportion of positive results that are truly positive. The negative predictive value is the proportion of negative results that are truly negative. Both positive and negative predictive values of screening instruments are expressed as percentages.

6) b.

The lifetime risk for a major depressive disorder in Western countries for women is one in four; for men it is one in ten.

7) c.

The annual incidence of schizophrenia worldwide is 10–20 per 100 000 population. Some studies have shown a higher annual incidence in some ethnic groups such as Afro-Caribbean immigrants in the UK.

8) d.

Suicide rates are highest in older men. The risk is higher if they are unmarried or divorced.

9) a.

Children brought up by a biological parent suffering from schizophrenia are likely to have a higher rate of schizophrenia than the general population.

10) b.

Incidence is a measure of the frequency with which an event, such as a new case of illness, occurs in a population over a designated period of time. The formula for calculating an incidence rate is as follows:

$$\text{Incidence rate} = \frac{\text{New cases occurring in a given time period}}{\text{Total population in a given time period}} \times 10^n$$

11) c.

Prevalence is the proportion of people in a population who have a particular disease (both new and existing cases) over a specified period of time.

12) e.

The number of people with a particular illness at any time during a particular time interval is period prevalence.

13) c.

Prevalence is the total number of cases (both new and old) in a given population during a specified period of time.

14) b.

This report provides the relative risk of relapse of psychosis after exposure to cannabis. It means that there is a 4.41 times higher risk of relapse of psychosis in those exposed to cannabis.

15) b.

The odds ratio of 5.44 means that the odds of people developing cognitive decline after a severe head injury is 5.44 times higher than the odds in the general population.

16) a.

The reliability of an instrument gives an idea of how consistent the results will be if the instrument was used by a number of people or at different time intervals. Sensitivity gives an idea of how accurate an instrument is.

17) d.

Proportional mortality is described as a proportion of deaths in a specified population over a period of time attributable to different causes. Each cause is expressed as a percentage of all the deaths and the sum of the causes must add to 100%. For example, according to figures from the USA, in 1987, suicide was ranked eighth among the causes of mortality, with a proportionate mortality of 1.5%, which means that among all the deaths reported within the USA in 1987, 1.5% of those deaths were caused by suicide.

18) a.
The primary difference between incidence and prevalence is in what cases are included in X. For incidence, X is restricted to new cases; for prevalence, X includes both new and pre-existing cases.

19) b.
Prevalence is based on both incidence and duration. If the incidence of the two cancers is similar then the difference in prevalence must reflect a difference in duration. Since cancer A is more prevalent than cancer B, its duration must be longer than that of cancer B. The two possible explanations for cancer B being of shorter duration could be either rapid recovery or rapid mortality.

20) d.
The odds ratio for this case-controlled study can be calculated by arranging the data in the following 2 × 2 table

	Cases	Controls	Total
Exposed	A = 50	B = 25	75
Unexposed	C = 50	D = 75	125
Total	100	100	200

Odds ratio = AD/BC = 50 × 75/25 × 50 = 3.0

21) e.
The numerator includes pre-existing cases, so we know we are dealing with prevalence rather than incidence. Both numerator and denominator are measured at a point in time (1 January 2010) so it is point prevalence rather than period prevalence.

22) a.
Screening instruments are used to detect common syndromes such as depression, anxiety and alcohol abuse. They are not useful in detecting uncommon syndromes.

23) b.
The scores on a rating scale can be used to determine inclusion and exclusion from a study.

24) b.
Cohort studies are longitudinal and not cross-sectional.

25) d.
Adequate selection of controls will minimize the possibility of bias. Effort after meaning is the recall bias that can occur in ill people looking for an explanation for their illness.

26) d.
The confounding variables are not on the causal pathway between exposure and disease.

27) a.
Case-controlled studies are observational studies.

28) b.
The BPRS (Brief Psychiatric Rating Scale) is used to measure positive symptoms in schizophrenia.

29) c.
A confounder can either be an independent risk factor or a protective factor for the disease.

30) b.
High reliability does not necessarily imply high validity.

31) a.
The validity of a diagnosis describes the extent to which it corresponds to a gold standard and can be assessed in comparison with a gold standard.

32) b.
The specificity is the probability of not diagnosing disease when it is absent.

33) e.
Schizophrenia is equally common in males and females.

34) c.
In schizophrenia, the rates from urban areas are usually higher than those from rural areas. According to social drift theory (Goldberg & Morrison 1963) men are more likely to drift into inner-city areas. Breeder hypothesis (social causation hypothesis by Castle et al. 1993) suggested that some environmental factors of aetiological importance in schizophrenia are more likely to affect those born into households of lower socioeconomic status and in the inner city.

Castle DJ, Scott K, Wessely S, Murray RM. Does social deprivation during gestation and early life predispose to later schizophrenia? *Soc Psychiatry Psychiatr Epidemiol* 1993; **28**: 1–4.
Goldberg EM, Morrison SL. Schizophrenia and social class. *Br J Psychiatry* 1963; **109**: 785–802.

35) c.
The probability of psychiatric disorder is increased if there is a family history of psychiatric disorder, but not likewise for delusional disorder and schizophrenia.

Munro A. Phenomenological aspects of monodelusional disorders. *Br J Psychiatry* 1991; **14**: 62–4 (Suppl.)

36) c.
Depressive disorder is more common in females generally but male first admissions continue to climb until the end of life, overtaking female first admissions at the age of 85. The point prevalence is higher in women. There is a higher incidence in those who are unmarried. Brown and Harris found that there is a higher prevalence in working-class women than in middle-class women.

> Brown GW, Harris TO. *Social Origins of Depression: A Study of Psychiatric Disorders in Women*. London: Tavistock Press, 1978.

37) e.
Lifetime risk in the general population is 0.6–1.1%.

38) e.
Suicide is also common in single and widowed people, and is associated with unemployment and retirement.

39) e.
Deliberate self-harm is also common in unemployed people and those living in overcrowded inner cities.

40) e.
There is a high degree of overlap in agoraphobia, simple phobia and social phobia. Individuals with major depression have a 9–15 times higher risk of developing agoraphobia and simple phobia. Around 25% of patients with phobias report alcohol abuse.

41) b.
All socioeconomic groups are affected.

42) b.
Early-onset generalized anxiety disorder (GAD) is more likely in females.

43) e.
There is a bimodal age of onset, with peaks occurring at ages 12–14 and 20–22 years.

44) a.
Prevalence increases with increasing parity; there is a higher prevalence in those women who have experienced natural menstrual cycles for a longer period of time (whose cycles are not modified with oral contraceptive pills and are uninterrupted with pregnancy).

45) b.
Puerperal psychosis is more associated with higher social class.

46) d.
There is a significant association with higher parental education, and it is higher in ballet and modelling schools.

47) e.
The prevalence of bulimia in adolescent and young adult females is approximately 1–3%.

48) b.
The prevalence of dementia is 5%, depression 13.5%, phobic disorders 10%, paranoid states 0.5%, and personality disorders 1%. The prevalence of dementia rises with age, doubling every 5.1 years until in the over-80s it is 20%.

49) e.
Onset of Huntington's disease occurs in childhood in 10–20% of cases.

50) e.
There is an increased risk of schizophrenia in first-degree relatives but the association is less than when compared with younger-onset schizophrenia.

Further reading

Gelder M, Harrison P, Cowen P. *Shorter Oxford Textbook of Psychiatry*, 5th edn. Oxford: Oxford University Press, 2006.

Greenhalgh T. *How to Read a Paper: The Basics of Evidence-Based Medicine*, 2nd edn. London: BMJ, 2001.

Lawry S, McIntosh A, Rao S. *Critical Appraisal for Psychiatrists*. Edinburgh: Churchill Livingstone, 2000.

Puri B, Hall A. *Revision Notes in Psychiatry*, 2nd edn. London: Arnold/ Hodder Education, 2004.

Simon Fraser University. Statistics and Actuarial Science, 2009. www.stat.sfu.ca.